Halbert Weidner, CO, DPhil

Grief, Loss, a~~nd Death~~
The Shadow Side of Ministry

Pre-publication
REVIEWS,
COMMENTARIES,
EVALUATIONS . . .

"**H**albert Weidner has done a superb job in blazing a trail for ministers and lay clergy of all denominations. Addressing both the practical aspects of ministry alongside the intricate personal and often very lonely road that pastors everywhere must face, Father Weidner has shone a light on what has been heretofore darkened by silence. It was not only refreshing, but very timely in my own case. As the founder of an independent ministry whose purpose is largely to deal with those that are suffering the transition through grief and loss, Weidner's wise insights are extremely appreciated. As it is also my job to train ministers for our pastoral work, I am very familiar with those lonely conflicts we face when we 'take up the cross' that are so eloquently addressed—those of in a position of tremendous responsibility, while at the same time cut off from much of the rest of the world in so many ways.

Being generally outside the accepted professional community while at the same time having to remain removed from the private sector as one that must necessarily stand ready to be all things to all people, ministers indeed face challenges that only one on the inside understands—and few seem to talk about.

Our ministry specifically works with people that are working through the deep grief that can be experienced through loss of pets, which is a highly underserved area of pastoral care. It is a grief no less real and no less intense for many than any other, but of course this specialized area of pastoral care leaves me even outside of the loop of support from much of the cleric community. So this book was like a welcome friend! I will refer to it often as well as recommending it to the chaplains in my own ministry. I highly recommend this book to anyone in this field of holy service or to anyone contemplating the spiritual life."

Reverend Sandra Shaw
Founder, Chaplain of the Pets Interfaith Christian Ministry, Chapel of the Fields

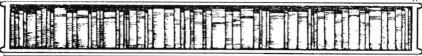

More pre-publication
REVIEWS, COMMENTARIES, EVALUATIONS . . .

"**I**n a clear and deep style, the author presents the basic realities faced by all ministers, regardless of their denomination. *Grief, Loss, and Death* deals with significant issues such as prayer, meditation, education, the family of the minister, grief, and many other important aspects of the ministry. The book presents the shadow side of ministry as 'our human selves'; and that human side of the minister is widely presented and discussed. This book should be read by any person involved in some kind of ministry. It will provide exciting dialogue and meditation, as well as hope, mission, and purpose."

Alfonso Valenzuela, DMin, PhD
Associate Professor of Pastoral Counseling and Marriage and Family Studies, Andrews University

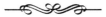

"**R**ight from the get-go, one understands that this small book is written from the personal experience of an intelligent heart and that it concerns the often secret or evaded matters of a full human life, feelings that call out for conscious reflection and prayer; namely, the deep personal sorrows and relationships, the dark issues, and the depression and the despair, that so readily insinuate themselves into the noonday sun of a life of total service to others.

Original, honest, and chock-full of psychological insight, each chapter begins with a story, a personal yet emblematic vignette, about the human wholeness that includes hidden shadows and the lonely dark. Stages, roles, and credentials, the professional and the legal sides of ministry, are perceptively contrasted and related to ministering from within the wisdom tradition, with its openness, dialogue, trust, and compassion. Not as a simple solution or escape, but as a sympathetic rendering of the experience of darkness as quintessentially human, the author offers the prayers of the liturgy, and Stations of the Cross, directly relevant readings, and the contrapuntal play of the Psalms with the words of Jesus—all as gracious counterparts to the eclipses of steadfast faith."

M. Katherine Tillman, PhD
Professor, Program of Liberal Studies, University of Notre Dame

The Haworth Pastoral Press®
An Imprint of The Haworth Press, Inc.
New York • London • Oxford

Grief, Loss, and Death
The Shadow Side of Ministry

THE HAWORTH PASTORAL PRESS®
Haworth Series in Chaplaincy
Andrew J. Weaver, Mth, PhD
Editor

Living Faithfully with Disappointment in the Church by J. LeBron McBride

Young Clergy: A Biographical-Developmental Study by Donald Capps

Grief, Loss, and Death: The Shadow Side of Ministry by Halbert Weidner

Prison Ministry: Hope Behind the Wall by Dennis W. Pierce

A Pastor's Guide to Interpersonal Communication: The Other Six Days by Blake J. Neff

Pastoral Care of Depression: Helping Clients Heal Their Relationship with God by Glendon Moriarty

Pastoral Care with Younger Adults in Long-Term Care by Reverend Jacqueline Sullivan

The Spirituality of Community Life: When We Come 'Round Right by Ronald P. McDonald

Pastoral Care from the Pulpit: Meditations of Hope and Encouragement by J. LeBron McBride

Grief, Loss, and Death
The Shadow Side of Ministry

Halbert Weidner, CO, DPhil

The Haworth Pastoral Press®
An Imprint of The Haworth Press, Inc.
New York • London • Oxford

For more information on this book or to order, visit
http://www.haworthpress.com/store/product.asp?sku=5157

or call 1-800-HAWORTH (800-429-6784) in the United States and Canada
or (607) 722-5857 outside the United States and Canada

or contact orders@HaworthPress.com

Published by

The Haworth Pastoral Press®, an imprint of The Haworth Press, Inc., 10 Alice Street, Binghamton, NY 13904–1580

PUBLISHER'S NOTE
The development, preparation, and publication of this work has been undertaken with great care. However, the Publisher, employees, editors, and agents of The Haworth Press are not responsible for any errors contained herein or for consequences that may ensue from use of materials or information contained in this work. The Haworth Press is committed to the dissemination of ideas and information according to the highest standards of intellectual freedom and the free exchange of ideas. Statements made and opinions expressed in this publication do not necessarily reflect the views of the Publisher, Directors, management, or staff of The Haworth Press, Inc., or an endorsement by them.

Identities and circumstances of individuals discussed in this book have been changed to protect confidentiality.

Cover design by Jennifer M. Gaska.

Library of Congress Cataloging-in-Publication Data

Weidner, Halbert.
  Grief, loss, and death : the shadow side of ministry / Halbert Weidner.
    p. cm.
  Includes bibliographical references and index.
  ISBN-13: 978-0-7890-2414-5 (alk. paper)
  ISBN-10: 0-7890-2414-4 (alk. paper)
  ISBN-13: 978-0-7890-2415-2 (pbk. : alk. paper)
  ISBN-10: 0-7890-2415-2 (pbk. : alk. paper)
  1. Church work with the bereaved. 2. Pastoral theology. 3. Death—Religious aspects—Christianity. I. Title.

  BV4330.W44 2006
  259'.6—dc22
                                                                    2005011227

CONTENTS

ABOUT THE AUTHOR

Halbert Weidner, CO, DPhil, is a teacher and pastor who has worked in various parishes, chaplaincies, and schools since he was ordained in 1974. His books include a critical edition of John Henry Cardinal Newman's *Via Media* and a pastoral book on spirituality, *Praying with John Cardinal Newman: Companions for the Journey.*

Preface and Acknowledgments

The noonday devil, despair, is the traditional enemy in ministry. *Grief, Loss, and Death* will help beginners prepare against allowing the situations they may face to bleach out all color and nearly all hope in their lives. Experienced ministers can use the book as a catalog to be consulted as despair tries to invade all their defenses. For those who are older and all the wiser now, perhaps this text will help them to arrange their memories.

Names and circumstances mentioned in the book have been changed to protect identity, except for the incomparable Liz Kekoa. Liz, who was killed in an accident, is well known in our area.

Special thanks to Maryknoll Father Cy Gombold. Cy Gombold was the first priest I ever knew and behind this text is my experience of him as the pastor who received me into the Catholic Church a long time ago. He was a good preacher, teacher, confessor, liturgist, and pastor. In an era when parish finances excluded the public and even the bishop, Father Gombold published the income and expenses report every year. He was also an alcoholic, although I don't remember a time when it interfered with his work. It did nearly destroy his ego, though. He thought his life was in ruins, but he was still faithful to love. He became a priest in the late 1960s when chaos was reigning after the Second Vatican Council. As the president of the priests' council he was the one all sides trusted. He died unexpectedly. At the funeral mass, the church was overflowing with mourners, even though he was new to the parish. Father Gombold had been demoted to assistant pastor, and had never been a sponsor of any organization. The people there were people whose lives he had touched, one by one. This book is for him and for the Maryknoll family.

Chapter 1

Stages of Growth
or the Stations of the Cross?

The shadow side of ministry shoots a bullet through the brain that does not kill or stop thinking or feeling. It does create a hole, a long, hollow, empty wound that thinking and feeling must somehow bypass. The wounded minister does not recover the previous self, cannot really remember what the old self thought or felt. As with a veteran of a secret war, there may be a new life after the shameful wound, but no public way to heal.

But there can be a public way of speaking about it and this may help relieve some of the shame and self-blame. Some of the shame comes from believing that the wound inflicted by the shadows was avoidable. True, a certain amount of chance is involved. Some in ministry may avoid or evade the shadow side altogether. The odds are against it. Luck favors the shadow side and not the minister trying to beat those odds. However, the biases of the enlightenment, its very name a weapon against shadows, tempt ministers into a reliance on rational, professional skills. So we must look at this first and obvious defense against the darkness imbedded in life. The weapons of the enlightenment prefer to speak about the positive growth that comes from encountering and mastering the challenges of human living. Ministers are supposed to know about these kinds of positive growth and be able to avoid loss.

People in ministry become experts on human growth. They know such growth comes in stages and they work patiently with people at different stages of growth. The different kinds of pastoral expertise that make this possible have come at a price. Professional knowledge has its price and a reward—degrees and certificates. Personal knowledge has its price, too. Both are sources, but

they do not always sit well together. They have different imperatives, strengths, and appeals. Studying "others" is one thing, but it
is another to know oneself. Professional knowledge cannot protect
the knower and when he or she knows this, something terrifying
yet great happens.

"Never let them see you sweat!" is an imperative used on the
professional side of pastoral care. "Clients" and parishioners would
be unnerved if they saw the price paid by pastoral ministers trying
to be attentive, empathetic, and professional. Another imperative
comes from the Gospel: "Take up your cross daily and follow
me!" (Luke 9:23 NIV). These two imperatives cross over and
make for double crossbearing. The imperative of the cross is about
the suffering servant. This tradition common to Jews and Christians offers a mysterious figure whose effectiveness comes from a
repulsive appearance and festering wounds. For Christians, this
figure can hardly be avoided even in churches where tradition bans
a crucifix. The professional who does not sweat knows that the answers and the suffering servant are incompatible, but the attempt
to glue the unglueable is human and ministers are human. So here
are humans trying not to be so human so they can help others be
human. This is not so much paradoxical as merely impossible.
Still we try. Many pastors, as do good doctors, hang professional
degrees on their office walls. Their clients don't know what they
went through to get those degrees but they feel sure such a professional status indicates sure and certain hands that won't sweat and
lose their grip. In the Stations of the Cross, a devotion centered
around pictures and the retelling of Jesus making his way from Pi-
late to death on the cross and burial, Jesus slips and falls three
times. This devotion, found in many Roman Catholic churches, is
an honest picture of what it means to be a minister who takes up a
cross. This is not to contradict the need for professionalism. Professionalism is necessary so that people are not injured by ignorance. But when it becomes gnosticism and promises a rescue
from being human, then it wounds the professional rescuer and
possibly the suffering already wounded.

The shadow side of ministry is simply the human side. The
shadow experience is the experience of limits, the very boundaries
of being a human, created and contingent. Theologically speak-

ing, it is the incarnational side. No incarnational academic degrees are required to be human. In fact, academia can be the innocent enemy of humanity, standing in for the tree of knowledge in the Garden of Eden. It is not so evil in itself, but it is inadequate for the task many want to give it: validation of human worth. This includes ministers facing situations that only God can handle. Faced with the impossible, we could say that the temptation in the Garden of Eden could get acted out in every pastoral situation. A tree of knowledge and a shortcut to the knowledge are present. The shortcut promises a God-like ability to work our way through good and evil. Those who come to ministers are half hoping that the minister is in fact not human but some kind of conduit of the Divine. We are, actually, but we are human conduits of the Divine and not a divine conduit. Even Catholics who believe that the Pope can be infallible as a teacher know that the Pope as a human being goes to confession and seeks absolution. There are no shortcuts for popes so why would anyone else attempt shortcuts or try to claim them or expect them? Of course, we could say, I am not a pope, I'm just a special me and claim an infallibility that would frighten off papal theologians and not a few angels.

The shadow side of ministry or the ministry of being human means that we really live outside what professional jargon calls "roles." Roles are shortcuts to identity. We do have roles, professional training, boundaries to observe, accountability, and requirements such as goals and some intentional means of getting there. But there is an energy required for these roles and this energy does not come from the role nor is it shaped by the role. The energy itself shapes the role. The energy has a personal shape that precedes the role and as such it can only come from the center of the person.

Fundamental to people is human nature. In school, human nature's task is simply to stay out of the way of learning. It is expected to stretch as far as the content demands, and be as flexible as professional methods require. In fact, if anything is inconvenient in academia, it is the very notion of human nature. For some academics, human nature is as archaic an idea as God. But even for those for whom God and human nature exists, the preference for a professional life with its social roles is present. The professional forum is public and one of standards. Here, the minister is judged. If that were the whole picture then the suffering servant of Isaiah would not pass the tests. In the human, shadowy side grace works and mystery thrives. Grace and mystery are notoriously shy of credentialing.

Credentials and public accountability are necessary, but they do not save. They do not save us because credentials do not bring us to God nor do they rescue us from suffering. The scandal of suffering in pastoral ministry comes to us who are schooled, accountable, and still not spared the role of suffering. When I was newly ordained, I joined a support group for ministers. I was the only Catholic priest. In the group were two saints. They had nearly fifteen years seniority on me, not to mention being well on their way to being canonized. Both were in serious trouble with their congregations, however. One had temporarily allowed a room in his church to be used by recovering drug addicts waiting for the city to finish their rehabilitation center. The other had fired a notoriously bad organist who was also related to half of the congregation. The beating these two men took for such "trivial" events gave me chills. I wondered what was going to happen to me, the green wood, if that is what happened to the dry. I knew I would always be in trouble in ministry. Perhaps both men had made poor decisions. I was naïve enough to think that their congregations, on the basis of their obvious goodness and generosity, would overlook the lapses. But this did not happen. Later I met the organist who was hired as the replacement of the mediocre one. She was fired by the pastor who came later. She was a fine musician but there had to be revenge. Part of the new minister's mandate was to make sure the offending replacement suffered the same fate as the organist had in the old regime.

Are these trivial events common? Yes; and the more painful because of that. Avoidable? We would all like to think so, at least in the beginning of our ministry. I was warned about such optimism by a friend whose sandwich franchise was failing. I wanted to support him in the business but the franchise offered a really poor product. Eating there was a sacrifice and not many people were up to it so bankruptcy for the shop was near unless the owner could find a buyer. And he did. I asked how that was possible. The owner said that there was always someone out there who thought he or she was smarter and that the problem with the shop was bad management. A confident person did come along and actually pay to take the shop off the hands of the first and desperate owner. Of course, the shop failed again, only this time the law of averages was against the owner and no one was foolish enough to try and be a rescuer. The owner went bankrupt. I have found this "they failed, but I won't" ideology in ministry. Yet the shadow side comes to us all. Some have failed in avoidable ways. The ineluctably tragic side of life comes even to the well-prepared disciple. The cross has always held precious gifts. Those who share a communion in suffering and in contemplation can find healing, meaning, and even joy if such well-disguised gifts can be received.

To say all this in professional jargon is to talk about "growth." Growth is an attractive metaphor. Descriptions of each stage of growth sound wonderful. Each individual stage has its own greatness. What is not so wonderful is the transition between the stages. Nobody I know has made the leap between one stage and the next, between one rewarding way of living to another level of reward. The move between stages is through the cross. Lack of faith is not what keeps some people from growing, but rather their native intelligence helps them naturally to avoid pain. Very often, it is unavoidable pain that drags us through the darkness and up to the next stage of development or we don't go at all. The instinct to resist, even by ministers and the congregations to whom they preach, can seem like common sense.

Paradigms of growth try hard to avoid delving into the dark nights of sense and soul that mediate the path. We can take an intellectual approach that draws a picture of ever-growing enlightenment and movement from the narrow and selfish to the universal and holy. The goal is attractive as long as the price tag stays hidden. Hiding the sticker price is the genius of gnosticism. It promises a concealed path perennially popular because it hides both the path and the cost of discipleship. The cross and its path are not secret. Much of the life of Jesus was secret, but not the cross. That degradation and the path to it were public. And the path for us is well marked, if narrow.

As a single person, for me the clarity of the way of the cross could not be brighter than in the lives of married couples who believe that their spousal relationship is sacramental. The path from a romantic beginning through disenchantment to a truthfully loving decision to remain married is a paradigm of the spiritual life. I recall a conversation I had with a woman on an Engaged Encounter team. She and her husband shared with other couples the pain their relationship had been through, almost ending their marriage. He was known as an exceptionally caring military officer whose men trusted him, maybe even loved him. But he was not as caring for his spouse as he was for his unit. The woman told me that Engaged Encounter communicated well certain stages of marriage moving from enchantment to disenchantment to love. But she said she believed that beyond disenchantment was something worse before love took over. Words failed her but she said it was more like living through hell. So maybe there is enchantment, disenchantment, hell, and then love. St. Silouan, the monk of Mt. Athos, said that the secret of the spiritual life was being able to stay in hell and pray. This woman's marriage difficulty taught her the wisdom learned by a hermit on a lonely mountain.

At workshops on the stages of the spiritual life, I discuss growth and maturity. The actual workshop content is about smelly messes. I take the materials from the desert tradition of John of the Cross and Teresa of Avila. John and Teresa know about the transitions between the stages. They are intellectually sound about the levels of growth and don't shrink from the blood and gore strewn in between. The desert tradition is old and realistic. It also intends to be healing without falling into a narcissism that other therapies sometimes encourage. The desert tradition trusts in reality as a kind of sacrament even when we are wounded. Unreality is slow poisoning. Unreality leaves us less in pain, but also less free. Unreality will slowly kill us and we know that because the comfort we feel comes from the soft wrappings of burial cloth being wound around us. We are dying or dead and are being gently treated.

Being called out of death by the ever-living One means having friends who roll the stone away, unwrap us, and set us free. We may not always thank the One who is life. We may resist the frightening noise of the rolling stone. Certainly the blinding light and the new nakedness that comes from being unswaddled cannot be comforting. Being born was not comforting and being born again is a shock. In both situations we thought that where we were—dark confinement—was our home.

In some traditions devotion consists of crosses with numbers and pictures that are mounted on the wall along the sides of the church. These are the Stations of the Cross. They depict events, some scriptural, some traditional, as Jesus carried his cross on his way to Calvary. The traditional movement is from the condemnation of Jesus to his burial. The climax is not the resurrection but the death of Jesus. To relieve the starkness, some churches add a resurrection station. Even then, this is a Christian exercise that contradicts the gnostic wish that suffering flesh stay out of spirituality. Suffering does not drive us into a zone of comfort with a God that helps us deny our limitations. Suffering is something that God takes part in. Why God wants to participate in our limitations has never been clear. It would be clearer if He wanted to save us from being creatures and shared the necessary knowledge that would rescue us. The shadow side of ministry is about being human because Jesus, Son of God, is human. The children of God always are.

The stages of our lives are more like Jesus in the Stations of the Cross than somebody's schema of stages of growth. We rise and fall and rise again on our way to an unavoidable death. We meet weeping and consoling friends and family, hostility, and mockery. We get assistance in carrying the cross and finally we are stripped of everything and die. Most of the world knows this, of course. They are not professionals and they did not go to school. The reality of the way of the cross does not keep them from going to weddings, having babies, playing, and creating. They know where they are headed, most sooner rather than later. If our professional ministry does not take their experiences into account, then it is not worth much professionally. We cannot comfort most of the world with the idea that death is natural and will come as just another stage in the circle of life when in fact it comes usually as an interruption. Often enough there is not time to learn the lessons of death since the way to it happens fast.

We don't need the morbid practice of keeping a human skull on the dining room table to get the picture of death and suffering nor must we jump into Yorick's grave and commune with his bones. But we do need to do something about our contemporary expectation that being professional or having professionals around will save us from the tattering of life.

The stages of growth that we are permitted to experience can give us some hints about what does save us. Since the stages include a periodic transition through hell, we might get used to the idea of dying and rising as a pattern. Different unearned crises in our lives can be the beginning of a sense of grace. When we feel we did nothing to bring on the problem and that we can do nothing to get out of it except to move in a clueless direction of surrender to hope, we gain an experience of actual grace. God knows why we have come to this station of life and He alone can lead us out. This is not passivity or clinging. This is surrender or floating on a stream of life and love greater than we are. Oppressed people who are suffering as victims of someone else's selfishness are not called to passivity. Even the great resisters (e.g., Gandhi or Martin Luther King Jr.) knew that the grace of resistance to evil comes from surrendering to unearned love.

As ministers in local communities or in hospitals, the one wisdom we can try to live and share is this wisdom of surrender. Surrendering to grace is the only issue of life because it is the only thing that can give life. Surrendering is the source of creativity and energy because what we surrender to is on our side. Saying that the One to whom we surrender is greater than us and this infinite gap causes blindness because it is too bright is not dehumanizing. Darkness is trusted because it is benign and humanizing.

Demonic leaders offer a false path that promises tremendous light in exchange for infantilizing their followers. The demonic tips us off by offering surrender and a clear program with well-defined rewards. They tell followers that the path can be known, the enemies conquered, and that even death can be chosen as a weapon. The sadness that leads their followers to murder or death is never given up. Instead, it is turned into a weapon.

The wisdom tradition teaches a surrender that transforms wounds but never turns anyone or anything into a weapon. Death is never turned into a chosen program. Left as a mystery, an interruption even, it is never permitted the false light of ideology. But the real threat to surrender does not come from demonic leaders who would bring down death on their followers. The real threat is leadership that brings down death on outsiders. Suffering imposed on others is the standard response to the threat of suffering to ourselves. Imposing suffering on ourselves for the sake of others is, despite St. Paul and the popularity at weddings and funerals of I Corinthians 13, not common. I Corinthians is realistic and not romantic despite its poetic rhythms. This is a description of the way of the cross, not the stages of a natural unfolding of human nature. The way of the cross is a sweaty and bloody affair, but so is the way of love, so is the way of being human.

So there are no shortcuts to being human. None of the stages can be skipped and skipping through the transitions and just landing full grown at each stage of life is not permitted. For many, there are more Stations of the Cross than stages to growth. However, the surrender necessary for birth and necessary for death is also necessary for the transitions of growth. Usually, we scramble to the next stage because the one we were standing on crumbled under us and we could not stay there anyway. We get our new stage in life, our next station along the way, whether we want it or not. This is not a very Western idea, and does not fit the rational and individualistic agenda of the age. It is a Christian idea and one that is shared with other wisdom traditions. This criticizes the notion that we are the captains of our souls and that God's ways are our ways.

Since there are no shortcuts, professional ministers should not be ashamed when all their academic credits do not add up to some kind of bridge out of human nature. We are where we are because of grace. Grace taught our hearts to fear, relieved that fear, and even, once upon a time, helped us to become professionals. Grace just wants us to know how much is a gift. Suffering and not knowing all the answers are as well.

Throughout this book, the image used of ministry is the *both/and* life that is central to the minister's vocation. The *either/or* is lived out at each stage of life, but the transitions are both/and and therefore, the prevailing image is the cross. The cross represents both/and. Jesus is suspended between heaven and earth on the cross. The suspension looks like hell and, indeed, he will descend into hell and only then will be there be Easter. But even on Easter, the wounds suffered in the suspension will not disappear. They will be transformed, but always a part of his identity. And so it is with people who minister.

Chapter 2

A Feast Day Funeral

After a death in the congregation, a parishioner asks, "How is the family taking it?" The casual brutality of that question is forgivable because of the ignorance of human suffering it displays. Other times or places the question would be unnecessary. "They" are wrapped in grief, moving in and out of numbness, overwhelmed by uncontrollable tears.

Current fashion allows for some grieving, but only if it does not go on for a long time. And a long time in some circles is a week! What drives this callousness is hard to say. Perhaps industrialization does not allow for grieving any more than it allows for pregnancy or child rearing. Something of the juice of life has passed away so life's mess is an obstacle to be overcome by bracketing. Some funerals are very clearly moments of hygiene, a disposal of a potentially disease-bearing trash that once was the body of a living person. The dead simply fall behind and we are a marching army so we cannot pay attention to them.

The minister in attendance to the dying and grieving can be expected to be professional and not invest in any of the emotions that used to be shared by the larger community. This is easy to do because the dead and grieving were only marginally attached to the community now entrusted with the disposal of the body. I cannot say burial anymore because cremation is becoming more and more popular. The various means of committing the ashes range from the secular and indifferent to solemn religious ceremonies common to Buddhism and now even found in Catholicism.

Many Protestant churches are small communities and the number of *active* Catholics is also small, even in large parishes. More often than not, the minister knew the person, maybe even loved him or her. The shadow side of ministry penetrates our defenses again.

Some ministers and staff may choose to "handle" funerals the way mechanics handle cars or even dentists take on tooth decay. These expectations can result in terrible dilemmas when scheduling must be done. In my own ministry an example came one May when our community was celebrating its founder, Philip Neri. An Italian saint of the Counter-Reformation in Rome, he was an extraordinarily cheerful and attractive person. He has been captured by the Oratorians he founded as the patron saint of joy. A few years ago the staff, following the limitations imposed by the funeral home who are in turn imposed upon by the people who open the graves, selected our feast day for a funeral.

The funeral was scheduled for the morning and the feast day celebrations in the evening. I was to preside at both, turning on a funeral switch and then a fiesta one. The funeral was for David, a young man who had committed suicide. So someone thought that what ministers do is minister to a family nearly unhinged by death and then turn to the feast day.

The following is the homily I delivered at the funeral. I am including it at this point because it was my way of dealing with the impossible task of trying to be joyful and present to deep sorrow at the same time. I rarely write out anything more than an outline, even for long homilies. But I wrote out every word of this one because I was afraid my memory would be overwhelmed when I faced David's family and friends.

> Today is the day my community celebrates the death of its founder, Philip Neri.
>
> He died an old man, surrounded by those he loved. He lived a long life for the time—eighty years old.
>
> His work has lasted in some form or another for 400 years. He is the patron saint of joy. What would this saint of joy, this Philip Neri, this man who lived to eighty, say to us today? He lived in hard times. He was with many who died young and even who died violently. The joy in his life was not gotten cheaply or quickly.

Certainly Philip was among the angels and saints who surprised and welcomed David home when David died.

What would St. Philip Neri say to us today?

He would, I think, beg us to anchor our hopes and joys in God alone—he would know that any other place is shallow to withstand the sorrows and terrors of this world.

So when we face the sorrow and terror of David's death, our hope is anchored in the promises of God.

David knew a terror and a sorrow that caused such pain, he knew no other way out. This pain has a medical name because it is a medical condition caused by chemicals raging in the body. He died from that as someone can die in a car accident or from cancer.

Our sorrow and terror in the face of such a death can make us forget that all of us are here—in the best of circumstances—for just a little while.

What saves us is not luck, or good health—all these are temporary—but the eternal love of God.

David knows that, St. Philip lived it.

We cannot have David back.

But we can live with the truth that we would tell him if we could have him back.

We would say to David: Love made us; Love sustains us; Love will not let us go.

God promised that, David, and you know that now that you are home with God.

I was able to go from this very sad funeral to the feast-day celebrations grounded in something deep and weighty but not contradictory to what the festivities called for. The wisdom tradition of spirituality says that authentic lives are lived on the razor's edge. The lives of the holy ones make us dizzy. Multiple versions of either/or are present here: joy/sadness, indifference/commitment, faith/despair, love/isolation, desire/compulsiveness—all the roads have forks in them. Some days we are called to live at the crossroads, under the cross, and be joyful without going down the road to joy just yet. The shadow side of ministry's sorrows intruding on ministry's joy can be born if we are not scandalized by the necessity of hope. Hope sees down the road over the horizon. If liturgy does not celebrate this, what does it celebrate?

Sorrow and joy, roughly placed together by circumstances, must be encountered more deeply by our liturgies. This does not lighten the shadow so much as to acknowledge it and to enlarge our hope for things not yet seen. For fifteen years our homilist at the community Christmas celebration has read the Christmas sermon from T.S. Eliot's *Murder in the Cathedral* (1971). As with most ministers, our scattered community cannot celebrate Christmas or any big feast day together. So, we designate the day after for the community gathering. The days after Christmas are bloody feasts: St. Stephen the Martyr, the Holy Innocents, and St. Thomas Becket, the martyred Archbishop of Canterbury. Eliot's play is about the murder of Thomas in the cathedral shortly after Christmas in 1170. The Christmas sermon of the archbishop written by Eliot exactly describes the great shadow and light partnership in the liturgy:

> Dear children of God, my sermon this morning will be a very short one. I wish only that you should ponder and meditate the deep meaning and mystery of our masses of Christmas Day. For whenever Mass is said, we re-enact the Passion and Death of Our Lord; and on this Christmas Day we do this in celebration of His Birth. So that at the same moment we rejoice in His coming for the salvation of men, and offer again to God His Body and Blood in sacrifice, oblation and satisfaction for the sins of the whole world.

> Not only do we at the feast of Christmas celebrate at once Our Lord's birth and death: but on the next day we celebrate the martyrdom of His first martyr, the blessed Stephen. Is it an accident, do you think, that the day of the first martyr follows immediately the day of the Birth of Christ? By no means. (Eliot, 1971, pp. 199-200)

The soon-to-be martyred archbishop says that a martyr is not just a good Christian who has been killed because of the faith. Such an event can only be mourned. Nor is the martyr simply a good Christian now made a saint. That would simply be to rejoice.

So thus as on earth the Church mourns and rejoices at once, in a fashion that the world cannot understand; so in Heaven the Saints are most high, having made themselves most low, seeing themselves not as we see them, but in the light of the Godhead from which they draw their being. (Eliot, 1971, pp. 199-200)

In the confrontation between sorrow and joy, mysticism is not an option, but a necessary step in spiritual development.

The power of this mysticism centers on the cross and is quite different from what mysticism is in the New Age. The crucified God of Christianity that we encounter at the crossroads holds before us the elements of our hope. In Matthew and Mark, we learn to pray Psalm 22, which begins with the crossroad experience of the rawest hopelessness: "My God, my God, why have you abandoned me?" Secular society lives without a God and without a question such as this. In the world of those who have lost faith, this question has been answered by a silence from God and consequently the withdrawal into silence by one who once believed enough to ask the question. An actor raised a Catholic was asked what would he say to God if there were a heaven and the actor got there. He replied, "You've got a lot of explaining to do!" The audience listening burst into applause.

For ourselves living for richer or poorer, in sickness and in health, married to a crucified God, the question of abandonment was one that was itself on the lips of the dying Lord. We pray it, but we pray it all the way through. One way to do this is pray the psalm with a challenging antiphon taken from Matthew 10:29, 31, NRSV: "Are not two sparrows sold for a penny? Yet not one of them will fall to the ground apart from your Father. So do not be afraid; you are of more value than many sparrows."

My God, my God, why have you forsaken me? Why are you so far from helping me, from the words of my groaning? O my God, I cry by day, but you do not answer; and by night, but find no rest.

Are not two sparrows sold for a penny? Yet not one of them will fall to the ground apart from your Father. So do not be afraid; you are of more value than many sparrows.

Yet you are holy, enthroned on the praises of Israel. In you our ancestors trusted; they trusted, and you delivered them. To you they cried, and were saved; in you they trusted, and were not put to shame.

Are not two sparrows sold for a penny? Yet not one of them will fall to the ground apart from your Father. So do not be afraid; you are of more value than many sparrows.

But I am a worm, and not human; scorned by others, and despised by the people. All who see me mock at me; they make mouths at me, they shake their heads; "Commit your cause to the Lord; let him deliver—let him rescue the one in whom he delights!"

Are not two sparrows sold for a penny? Yet not one of them will fall to the ground apart from your Father. So do not be afraid; you are of more value than many sparrows.

Yet it was you took me from the womb; you kept me safe on my mother's breast. On you I was cast from my birth, and since my mother bore me you have been my God. Do not be far from me, for trouble is near and there is no one to help.

Are not two sparrows sold for a penny? Yet not one of them will fall to the ground apart from your Father. So do not be afraid; you are of more value than many sparrows.

Many bulls encircle me, strong bulls of Bashan surround me; they open wide their mouths at me, like a ravening and roaring lion.

Are not two sparrows sold for a penny? Yet not one of them will fall to the ground apart from your Father. So do not be afraid; you are of more value than many sparrows.

I am poured out like water, and all my bones are out of joint; my heart is like wax; it is melted within my breast; my mouth is dried up like potsherd, and my tongue sticks to my jaws; you lay me in the dust of death.

Are not two sparrows sold for a penny? Yet not one of them will fall to the ground apart from your Father. So do not be afraid; you are of more value than many sparrows.

For dogs are all around me; a company of evildoers encircles me. My hands and my feet have shriveled; I can count all my bones. They stare and gloat over me; they divide my clothes among themselves, and for my clothing they cast lots.

Are not two sparrows sold for a penny? Yet not one of them will fall to the ground apart from your Father. So do not be afraid; you are of more value than many sparrows.

But you, O Lord, do not be far away! O my help, come quickly to my aid! Deliver my soul from the sword, my life from the power of the dog! Save me from the mouth of the lion. From the horns of the wild oxen you have rescued me. I will tell of your name to my brothers and sisters; in the midst of the congregation I will praise you: You who fear the Lord, praise him! All you offspring of Jacob, glorify him; stand in awe of him, all you offspring of Israel! For he did not despise or abhor the affliction of the afflicted; he did not hide his face from me, but heard when I cried to him.

Are not two sparrows sold for a penny? Yet not one of them will fall to the ground apart from your Father. So do not be afraid; you are of more value than many sparrows.

From you comes my praise in the great congregation; my vows I will pay before those who fear him. The poor shall eat and be satisfied; those who seek him shall praise the Lord. May your hearts live forever!

Are not two sparrows sold for a penny? Yet not one of them will fall to the ground apart from your Father. So do not be afraid; you are of more value than many sparrows.

All the ends of the earth shall remember and turn to the Lord; and all the families of the nations shall worship before him. For the dominion belongs to the Lord, and he rules over the nations.

Are not two sparrows sold for a penny? Yet not one of them will fall to the ground apart from your Father. So do not be afraid; you are of more value than many sparrows.

To him, indeed, shall all who sleep in the earth bow down; before him shall bow all who go down to the dust, and I shall live for him. Posterity will serve him; future generations will be told about the Lord, and proclaim his deliverance to a people yet unborn, saying that he has done it.

Are not two sparrows sold for a penny? Yet not one of them will fall to the ground apart from your Father. So do not be afraid; you are of more value than many sparrows.

The end of the psalm celebrates the light that God and the holy ones bring to us. We are not only united to God but to the whole assembly. Isolated from God and despairing of even relationships, we come into the heart of He who holds the hearts of all. We begin with an isolation that unbelievers think cancels out God and we end with a sense of grace and union with Him. We can ask God to forgive even our killers, to grant them dying next to us a paradise not even the best can imagine, and to render back to the God whose spirit breathes in us all the breath that is more dependent on the Creator than it is on healthy lungs.

The vocation of the minister is to keep the sorrow and the joy before a people who live in a culture that cannot face its own despair. It makes do with sad falsehoods such as, "She is not really dead because she will always live in our hearts." Such a statement is not just sentimental and false but covers despair with only the thinnest of veneers.

Grieving itself, even for those experiencing the greatest loss, is acceptable only for a short period of time. Oh, their son died? How are they taking it? Well, to tell the truth, they are in a fetal position as if they were kicked in the stomach by a horse and won't be in the office today or making the rounds or keeping any appointments. This might be acceptable for a short time, but not for long.

If some ministers do not believe that the culture evades sorrow, they will find out just how far the culture is willing to go when grief comes to the ministers themselves. The display of our own grief will be considered as a betrayal of our "function." A community is unsettled by the visible grief of its minister. But ministers are not allowed to grieve over their parishioners, their clients, the "objects" of their pastoral care. That would get in the way of serving them. So a minister should be able to switch from task to task without registering the cost. For some, this means they willingly take up their job as "a role" and move from role to role and then go home relatively pleased by the rewards of an objective measure of effectiveness. Personal investment and personal cost are neither part of the measure nor of the effectiveness. "Can't handle a funeral and wedding in the same day, what's your problem? A funeral on your day off, what's the problem? It only takes an hour." The minister can accept this value, hide the grief, get sick, or he or she can minister from the grief.

One task of a spiritual companion is to allow the minister to grieve over small and large losses. The people who seek ministering will discount totally the small griefs and perhaps allow a little time for the great ones. Surrounded by grief, the time for a minister to grieve must be more public and longer than allowed for by public expectation. A minister that ignores personal grief out of a sense of professionalism might be convinced to grieve more if there were a sense that grief is a source of better ministry than power and control. If we hang a diploma on the wall indicating our professional credits, we could hang another parchment from the school of hard knocks. This school has helped us to recover from a common lie used to motivate young people: "Work hard, keep your nose clean, and you will be rewarded." That this is not the Gospel and certainly not always true is a fact that we learn by experiencing the stripping of our egos by circumstances. In those circumstances, providence provides us with the material to reach out to other creatures, great and small, all of whom are going to die, returning to the dust. Our fragile fidelity is what God wants and our solidarity with creation. Knowing that salvation does not mean being spared the common lot must be a powerful source of ministry because it unites and grounds us in reality.

Chapter 3

Rod and Staff: Co-Workers

In the middle of an early Sunday morning Mass, I was handed a note saying that I should call the trauma unit of the city hospital. I handed the note to the sacristan who left to make the phone call. After Mass, we learned that our do-everything pastoral worker, Liz Kekoa, had been in an accident and might be dead. I focused on might be dead because early in my ministry I had been told about a death that never happened and I didn't want to go through that double shock again. I called my associate pastor and he took the next Mass and I went with staff to the hospital. On the way we saw the Kekoa van abandoned, wrecked, surrounded by police on the other side of the freeway. When we got to the hospital, Liz was indeed dead. I was the first to see her lying there lifeless, with only a small cut on her forehead, her hair neatly in place. She died from a broken neck. A young man racing on the freeway had caused the accident. He was a graduate from a local Catholic school and a schoolmate of her son. The courts were unable to legally determine who was at fault. We had to suffer both Liz's death and the long delays of the legal system. "Justice delayed is justice denied" does not seem to be an operating principle. Finally, the young man pleaded "no contest" to a charge of negligent homicide.

As Liz had done so many times alive, she called us to prayer. I could barely get through the beautiful prayers for the dead in our book of rites. We surrounded her body, trying to support one another and encircle the woman we had lost. We sobbed, choking back tears. An hour later, I had to go to her husband, hospitalized upstairs in a neck brace, and tell him that Liz was dead.

From time to time in these instances, a young clinical pastoral trainee would join us. As we waited for some paperwork to be filled out, this trainee took me aside, I believe to be of some consolation. She said to me, "It is really difficult to separate two different roles." I cannot remember what I said, but I was stunned. My "role" as a pastor and my "role" as a co-worker and friend was what I think she was talking about. She was using professional jargon and being graded on her ability to make such categories work. But she might have been a sociologist from another planet. Roles? Roles are for plays and movies. This was life and I was there because I loved Liz first and foremost and not because I was there to play my part.

It is difficult to explain to people that ministry is not a role. Have I ever questioned the role of the ministry? I have rejected the idea that ministry is a role. A role would allow me to function without pain, without personally extending my core. Ministry as a "role" is like being a doctor who cannot be both a good doctor and be personally involved. This rejection of person in favor of role is based on something that favors objectivity as an ideal way of dealing with people. But if we are objective, could we say that what people need and want is love and not "objectivity"? Could we not say that loving is a real way to know? Objectivity makes an object out of the person who ministers and the one who is ministered to. Does my crying while praying cancel out the prayer? What is the purpose of a priest standing by the dead if the priest is there as some kind of totem? We can comfort others while we grieve ourselves. What kind of "role" is that? What kind of comfort?

An even deeper question was why was I grieving? I loved Liz but she was in my life as a co-worker, not a friend. She was part of the mission and valued the same things I valued and was ready to do the work of five people to get the mission moving. In church work as in most places, co-workers are in place accidentally but can be lovingly received. They do not share secrets or a social life with us, but they know a secret part of us that our family and friends do not. They see us more than family and friends and we live with them in a special, in-between place with its own great light and sorrows.

Trying to explain the in-between stages of anything is really trying to explain a mystery. In evolution, for instance, how did we get from non-life to life? How did we get from the non-conscious to the conscious? How did we get from the fundamentally determined to the fundamentally free? The ordinary world had plenty of in-between stages that are closed to us now. Now we experience things as either/or. But once upon a time, the ordinary world in all its diversity depended on a both/and stage that bridged realities. The social world has its either/or structures and its both/and realities. In the social world, theorists say that there are organizations that are personal and organizations that are business. One is called a "gemeinshaft" and another "gesellschaft." One is about me and mine, the other is about selling. One organization is self-chosen and personal; the other is accidental and professional.

Ministry is not done in an either/or kind of world, but a both/and lifestyle that energizes diversity. The ministry team is one of those in-between realities that is hard to find in real life. Ministry has professional standards and measures, salaries and salary scales, taxes and benefits. This is not a description of the elements of friendship. These professional structures do not finally define ministry. Ministry is more than the grammar of business. Its energy depends on more than the structures. Inside the structure are people sharing something very rare: common values and dedication to a task for its own sake. Although co-workers are different than friends, they are not less than friends. We spend more time with co-workers than we do with family and friends. More important, our ministry, a life's project, is deeply affected by our co-workers. What family, friends, and co-workers in ministry have in common is the deep quality of their call to self-transcendence in ministry.

If by some miracle you were given the choice of either getting a new friend or a new dedicated co-worker, which would you choose? The choice is not easy. Since we spend more time with co-workers than we do with friends, co-workers have more power over our daily lives than most friends. The business world has its own fairly impersonal dynamic: in the *Godfather* people are murdered by associates for business reasons, not "personal" ones. Ministry is about a staff that builds on personal relationships. This does not mean evaluations and audits are out of order, but once accountability has been established, in fact, cherished by energetic, creative co-ministers, personal relationships begin to flourish somewhere between the lines of friendship and professional task forces. Friends may or may not be supportive of the ministry we find as our central project in the world. Although friends may provide consolation after-hours during a difficult ministry, many people would pass up the need for consolation in the first place and choose a supportive co-worker.

Liz Kekoa epitomized for me the miracle of a co-worker in mission. I could not say anything better about this than I did at her funeral:

> If there was anyone ready to go home to God then it was Liz Kekoa. She was part of a company of holy women who from the beginning have made the works of faith possible. If there was an Abraham, there was a Sarah. If there was an Isaac, there was a Rebecca. If there was a Jacob, there was a Rachel.
>
> For Jesus there was Martha and Mary and the home they with their brother Lazarus provided for Jesus. For Jesus there was Mary Magdalene with whom he entrusted the Easter proclamation of faith, the apostle who brought the good news to the apostles.
>
> For Jesus and his disciples there is the famous short list of women who followed them and provided for the ministry: Mary Magdalene again, Joanna, Susanna, and many other anonymous women "provided for them out of their own resources." (Luke 8:1-3, NRSV)
>
> And for us there was Liz Kekoa.
>
> There is no mission of the Church without these holy women.
>
> How is this possible? Liz was not a priest. Not a deacon. She was supposed to be without power. But powerful she was. There is only one power despite all the foolish weak things of this world masquerading as power and that is God's power and God's only power is the power of love. Liz had that power.
>
> How is this possible? Liz was only a human being. And human beings are not perfect and Liz was not perfect. But holi-

ness has nothing to do with perfection; it has to do with love. Liz did not wait to become perfect before she risked loving.

Liz was also wise. She had a habit of saying, "Welllllll, youuuuuuuuuuuuuuu know . . ." and she would stop. She would make those three words a complete sentence. She relied on you to know, to understand, to accept, and then to do the right thing. She was wise and she thought you were wise, too.

Liz was of great faith. If anyone had the right to lie down and give up, she had that right. She did not. Only the Holy Spirit could give someone that energy and only a great faith can receive that energy from God.

But to remember all this is a dangerous thing for us. Our wisdom tradition reminds us that to remember anyone with love is itself a call to action. What good would it do if we remembered and grieved for Liz without doing the works Liz thought were important?

Dearest to Liz's heart was the Jesus who welcomed the children. She invited, cajoled, bribed people (bribed them with heaven) to help her with sacrament preparations, Sunday school, youth ministry. She was passionate about ministry to children who did not attend parochial school, she loved our parochial school, its principal, staff and teachers, and children and gave herself to teaching religion every day. Liz believed in God's work for the young. She was willing to be an instrument of God's work for them. To replace her would take at least five people. Liz would say, "Why not ask for fifty people . . . for five hundred people . . . you know I was just getting started . . . we need all those people."

We needed Liz, and many more like her. May she in the communion of saints still join us in prayer every day so God our Father can work on our hearts and we can take up where she left off. May this loving God make us his imperfect people, perfect examples of what weakness can do with God's love just as God did for Liz.

When we experience co-workers as dedicated and supportive of our mission something very deep happens: our co-workers share our values and measure up to high standards. This makes us feel less lonely in a world with different standards and values. This is especially true in ministry where the usual career payoffs are lacking. Power and money in ministry are usually more marginal and we are less afraid of being manipulated by false intimacy and affirmation than, say, businesspeople would be. Structures and budgets are not easily reshaped regardless of our relationships within the staff. More love is at stake than money or power.

Of course, the major exception here in ministry includes those church and administrative positions where real power is a factor. When power is an important component in a particular ministry, the minister is usually isolated from real relationships within the ministry structure and becomes intimate only with family and friends on the outside. Ministries of power draw the minister into a circle of fear, especially of manipulation, so most people in these positions choose distance from colleagues even if it means a serious breach in community. The emotional cost to the minister is enormous. The blight can spread as the safety zone around the power is enlarged to include family, and most especially, spouses. The spouse can be given a public role of "special friend," but often the spouse is at risk in the relationship. Divorce among ministers and emotional isolation of celibate bishops and priests is too common.

Francis of Assisi could be a brother to everyone because he had no power and no possessions. People could get close to him because he had nothing they could take and no power to delegate. The pope that approved Francis and his rule of life could not be anyone's brother. He was surrounded by advisors, many of them hoping to outlive and replace him.

When power is inherit in a ministry, the give-and-take of relationships is lost. When someone in authority asks down the chain of command, "What do you think?" the person "below" hears the question as, "Do you want to keep your job?" and responds appropriately. The office space for ministries involving power might as well be located at the North Pole for all the intimacy—and honesty—that can be invited there. It is a cost that ministries without power do not demand.

Few people minister with much power. In fact, if providence operates at all in the lives of ministers it is through circumstances created through relationships within the team. We have experienced different directions in our life choices, but only some of these have been due to isolated personal decisions. The presence or absence of certain colleagues has been at least as important as our own private agenda.

For sure, we have experienced the loss of options when certain colleagues were lost. Some died, some moved away, some resigned. But because of this, by a certain age, we realize our life was deeply impacted by their absence, and perhaps for the worse. A path closed when a co-worker died or resigned. This same thing can happen in politics or business, but it is different in ministry. The influential co-worker was not there because of a power play or manipulation, but was there in the way of ministry, a way of shared values and sacrifices. The relationship was a gift outside of strategy; the way closed was a dream about service. After awhile we can carry more than a small number of regrets not because of poor moral or strategic decisions, but simply through the loss of a vision foreclosed by losses beyond our control.

Although we may not actually socialize with most of the team or staff, we spend most of our time with them and receive and give an energy that family and friends may know little of. In fact, a good co-worker can relieve the intrusion of family upon the ministry just as family can provide support when ministry is rough. So the presence of good co-workers is deeply valued; their absence deeply felt; their departure or worse, their death, profoundly mourned.

We can look at various staff situations and see the cross and the grace it invites. When the ministry team has the energy of love and mutual regard to draw on, the team will also be invited into the mystery of the cross and suffering. Some of the experiences of staff can be described as breakdowns and breakups. The intrusion of the shadow among staff can make ministers feel abandoned and isolated.

When a staff member breaks down, this is a disaster. First of all, it is not supposed to happen and there is the cold slap of scandal. The scandal comes because we somehow projected perfection. We wanted people to trust us and a cheap and short way to do this is paint ourselves and our colleagues as people without serious faults.

Professional standards are there as much to protect an image as to provide work standards. Professionalism is one way to hide perfectionism. In this case perfectionism has failed, as it must, and professionalism has not stopped the failure, as it was supposed to. We fail to include in our professional image the necessity of dealing with failure and the forgiveness and reconciliation that must follow. We bounce between coddling failed ministers and flaying them alive.

The current tendency is to flay. Outsiders say that the church is the only army that shoots its own wounded. On battlefields chosen by the church, there are no death-defying rescues of wounded colleagues. The lawyers discourage it, the hierarchies and judicatories won't defend compassion among the lower ranks, and all that stuff that is preached about forgiveness and reconciliation is carefully fenced off from the preachers. The minister is left with the impression that grace can be preached only by those who do not need it. The only acceptable minister does not experience the need for grace and has kept shame at bay with good behavior. If he or she has not, then good-bye.

In Roman Catholic circles, a certain archbishop got involved with a woman and fathered a child. Church money was used for supporting this clandestine family. Of course, the archbishop was out. But I remember ordinary parishioners who saw the good in the archbishop and wanted him back after he apologized. After all, they said, he repented and we are Christians, so why not? Before the Vatican II Council in the 1960s, there were what was known as "silent" priests. They got into trouble with money, or alcohol, maybe a consensual sexual relationship. They would be assigned a parish but had no permission to preach or hear scheduled confessions. Another priest would deliver mass. However, they could hear confessions if someone came to the rectory and asked for them. Very often, they were extremely popular confessors. Everyone knew that if they went to them for confession, there would be no scolding. The confessor had messed up and that was the kind of confessor many people wanted.

Resources are lost, not to mention the Gospel, when repentant ministers are cast out. In the Catholic Church, they are urged to live a life of prayer and penance and this has some merit, at least of giving worth to contrition. It would be strange indeed, if in the order of grace, much of the church was kept together by the humiliation and austere lives of the repentant. The ninety-nine might be saved by the one lost who did not forget being in the ninety-nine once and knew that more was needed than his or her own righteousness to be saved. Isolating the offenders from the community is more cruel than making them wear a red letter and keeping them as a brother or sister.

The false moralizing that justifies the expulsion of sinners from the ministry gets exposed when we consider a terrible fact: that besides ignoring fallen colleagues, the sick and dying also get ignored. We have a hard time facing limitations. A sick or dying co-worker, for example, challenges that inability and exposes our fear of the cross. I knew a dying priest with two good priest friends from decades past. I could not get the friends to come to the dying man's side. "He will only linger," said one of them to me as an explanation for an ill-timed departure leaving me and a couple of others to keep vigil through the night until the priest died. Some people will work for an organization that ministers to the suffering and then get caught in suffering because they care for their fellow ministers. Who ministers to suffering ministers who are suffering because their fellow ministers are suffering? What ministers will call for outside help when they are supposed to help others cope with this? Should such suffering be avoided by the ministers keeping their distance from one another? What is the painful shadowy side of supportive co-workers in the ministry? In a word, life's real problems intrude here because staff relationships can and do feed real life. Our reality is ministry and a supportive co-worker is not just a staff or business partner. When the blessing of a co-worker turns into the blessing of a cross, we can evade the grace it is trying to communicate in darkness.

This book is not about solutions or coping, but living through the shadow side. The death or illness of a co-worker who had supplied us with life can be lived through and not evaded. The relationship is itself the path to take. Our co-worker needs some space to communicate. I say communicate because it may not be through talking that the communication takes place. We can read these communications when we are with families that are the object of our ministry; we are not so prone to read them among our own colleagues. The closeness we feel to a co-worker in ministry needs to be explored because there are few parallels in the other worlds around us and few models for a minister.

Voluntary departure from the ministry challenges us just as breakdowns and breakups do. Everything said about the strange in-between intimacy of the ministry staff is underscored in feelings akin to divorce when valued co-workers depart for their own personal reasons. One word captures the sense of isolation: rejection. The departing co-worker has not only rejected the transcendent meaning of the mission that guides the lives of those left behind, those left behind feel their own persons violated when the ministry circle is broken.

A key moment for the community is the transition out of the circle. The departing minister can be treated as a traitor and even communications necessary for making the transition work can be cut off. Here, a professional sense could save the ministry. Professionalism could save the personal and transcendent by making the co-workers put the mission first and the ego damage second. Egos must be healed but they must not be in control.

The departure of a colleague highlights the perennial challenge of balance in ministry, the balance of a both/and vocation. The balance (and it is delicate as all balances are) is between the energy we get from the intimacy of staff relationships and the fear of losing our edge and compromising the mission by depending on the relationships. Perhaps the first time we realize this comes with the experience of the pain of loss at the departure of a staff person. We are professional ministers. Professional standards should make the staff interchangeable or the individuals less important. But we know this does not happen in a both/and organization. For the sake of the energy that comes from the personal, sometimes people must find their energies in something less personal. In treating departing colleagues and, really our own souls, fairly, we must pull back and simply follow procedures anointed by professional accountability.

The change of staff requires new kinds of relationships made more difficult by grieving over the lost colleague. The new colleague will face a special challenge. He or she will initially be seen as someone who has broken into the circle. This person is in the circle because it broke down, not because he or she was initially wanted. New colleagues are the both/and people in a both/and organization. They are not outside, but they are not inside. They replaced someone who was the center of some kind of trauma. If the new person has some kind of authority and his or her predecessor was well liked, that authority may be undermined as a memorial to the trauma. Not to undermine the new person would seem like a betrayal of the person who was replaced and a betrayal of the suffering the replacement caused. Many people must keep suffering going as a kind of memorial. This is a twisted love of the cross and of shadows. This ministry is half in love with easeful death. Preaching despair disguised as suffering love is easy. Easter did happen and although the shadow side of ministry can dominate, it cannot define. When the shadow side defines we call it despair. Recognizing when we are preaching despair disguised as hope is difficult.

Despair sets in when the both/and sides of ministry collapse. The ministry gives up both relationships and professional accountability. We choose not to relate to the new person or see how badly this affects the ministry we claim is all-important. At least a part of the ministry breaks down if not all of it. Dysfunction is another name for despair and in ministry it is not just a psychological or organizational problem, but a matter of faith. Faith energizes and reconstructs both polarities of ministry. Accountability saves us from being cruel because we are personally hurt. Relationships keep us from being cruel because we do not want to risk the bonding that shared values always invite. The relationships in ministry are, as noted earlier in this chapter, an invitation to self-transcendence. Transcending our grief is part of this, not as a way of denying the loss, but as a way of confirming that the lost relationship was for the sake of growth and a constant reaching out to others as a religious value. Jumping in an open grave and waiting for the earth to be piled on top of us is no memorial to the dead or departed. Ash Wednesday is a reminder to grow and change, not cringe and reject. We are all returning to dust and that is a liberating reality.

Chapter 4

The Death of Dialogue

Pressed between right-wing talk shows and left-wing political correctness I was not feeling at home anywhere and was getting nostalgic for my college days when Martin Buber's *I and Thou* (1971) and Reuel Howe's *Miracle of Dialogue* (1963) defined my expectations and responsibilities. Both books could not seem more marginal to my life today. I aked my Israeli friend Isaac if he knew Buber and what impact he had had on his life. Buber had been born in Vienna and died in Israel. *I and Thou* was very popular in the 1960s and fueled unrealistic hopes for a nation or at least a commune where people would not treat each other like objects— I-it.

To my surprise, Isaac had warm feelings for Buber and did not think him utopian. Isaac felt that what Buber wanted to see done in dialogue was getting accomplished still today in Isaac's work with foreign students coming to Israel. Isaac is a wonderful teacher with a great gift of languages: Polish, German, Hebrew, Spanish, French, English, and Russian. He is a Polish Jew, the only survivor in his family of Auschwitz. He illegally migrated to Palestine after World War II and took part in the Israeli-Arab war. He was left for dead outside the walls of Jerusalem, hearing the medics say, "This one won't make it" as they popped off his dog tags. Months later at attention with battalion at a memorial service for their dead, he heard his name read off! This man still believes in dialogue and I could not argue with him. Isaac continues to work today for peace and for living with the Palestinians. He has been attacked by nationalist Israelis and told he was encouraging another holocaust by trying to accommodate Palestinians.

Isaac and his wife Anna model for me a kind of supernatural natural goodwill that embraces life with both arms, giving and receiving warmth and energy. This does not mean that there are no arguments or misunderstandings. One really big one was the role of the Vatican during World War II and I pointed out that the pope helped by not condemning Stalin and allowing an enemy of the church to be an ally in the war with Hitler. Isaac had been an ardent socialist and yelled, "Forget Stalin!" What a funny moment! I have never heard anyone try to win an argument by saying Stalin was not important to World War II.

Isaac and Anna provide people with a hospitable place to have disagreements. The place is between the Old City of Jerusalem and Palestinian territory just to the south in Bethlehem, making their efforts very special. Their neighborhood has not been spared random acts of terrorism. Their grown children, dropping me off by the New Gate at the edge of old Jerusalem, told me that they never go into the old quarter, a place I roamed when the intifada was in full swing.

From this home on the border of war and terrorism, Isaac and Anna work with fellow Israelis and foreigners in the unending search for a way out of a spiral of violence. There, the choice of dialogue is the only choice for peace. Aggressive speech and acts of violence are the choices leading to perpetual war.

Holocaust survivors, the victims of the Shoah, remain irreducible miracles to me when they survive as lovers of humanity. I remember one woman in particular, a psychologist and a Jew from Czechoslovakia. She and her mother were arrested and transported in cattle cars to the concentration camp late in the war when there was no effort to disguise the place as anything but dying grounds. Corpses were lying around along the track and on the campgrounds. Both made a private vow not to die in front of the other. The violence in the camp reached a particular point of horror when one of the women gave birth to a baby boy. The guard seized it and in front of the women, drowned it under a spigot, saying, "Well, little Moses, you won't survive this time." The camp was liberated when the women were down to one bowl of greasy water per two people a day. She said that she and her mother shared the bowl and that after awhile she noticed that the liquid did not go down any after her mother pretended to sip. They both survived. When they and the other women were brought into the local German town to be processed out by the Red Cross, a German woman went by the ground floor windows pushing a baby carriage. The women rushed out to kill her baby. The psychologist ran out to push them back and with the help of the American army chaplain managed to save the woman and her baby. The chaplain said to her, "How did you preserve love all that time in the camp?" She replied, "I didn't preserve love, love preserved me."

Witnesses must surely hold us back in our personal crusades to disarm, strip, and morally destroy our opponents in the culture wars. Everyone seems to be a Nazi to everyone else. If Jesus came not for the righteous but the sinner, he would find few sinners around. Those without sin regularly try to stone to death the designated sinner du jour or, at least, deny tenure.

Ministry in the culture wars is overshadowed by the abandonment of dialogue. The substitution of rhetoric, euphemism, ad hominen logic, propaganda, and ideology, makes life simpler but ministry nearly impossible. People are canceled out as people and turned into objects to be resisted. It is war by other means. Killing others is not necessary if we can reify and transform them into things.

Henri Nouwen resurrected a piece of John Henry Newman's Anglican preaching to analyze the dynamic of resisting dialogue and its impact on religion. For some this is now a cliché but it is still fresh and new to others. The following is an eminent Victorian preaching at Christmas more than a century ago:

> Perhaps the reason why the standard of holiness among us is low, why our attainments are so poor, our view of the truth so dim, our belief so unreal, our general notions so artificial and external is this, that we are not trust each other with the secret of our hearts. We have each the same secret, and we keep it to ourselves, and we fear that, as a cause of estrangement, which really would be a bond of union. (Newman, 1899, pp. 126-127)

Then, as if this were not startling enough for the 1830s, he said:

> We do not probe the wounds of our nature thoroughly; we do
> not lay the foundation of our religious profession in the
> ground of our inner man; we make clean the outside of things;
> we are amiable and friendly to each other in words and deeds,
> but our love is not enlarged, our bowels of affection are strait-
> ened, and we fear to let the intercourse begin at the root; and,
> in consequence, our religion viewed as a social system, is
> hollow. The presence of Christ is not in it. (Newman, 1899,
> pp. 126-127)

If this was true at a time of polite enough discourse, what of today?
The short-circuiting that passes for argument today not only cuts
off thought but also people and not just the people attacked, but the
attackers, too. If people are attacked so is God.

Newman says that the lack of dialogue is a cover for shame and
guilt. Shame and guilt for what? Are we not passed that? No, it is
the guilt of being human and since the time of Genesis, the last
thing we want is to be human. Ideology promises transcendence at
no personal cost. We all become self-chosen prophets coming
down from the mountain with our commandments written on
stone. They are our commandments, not God's, and we toss the
stone tablets on a camp of the ungrateful who have better things to
do than conform their lives to our rules.

According to some polls (Gallup, 2005) we all believe this is
true, but we believe that it is our neighbor who does this, not us.
Results of one poll showed that roughly 80 percent of Americans
believe they live an ethical life and 80 percent believe that their
neighbors do not. How to do ministry in this kind of river of self-
righteousness? If I were a religious CEO I would make it a goal to
get those numbers down to 20 percent. It would not be hard if we
could agree on the wounds of our nature that we all hold in common and try to hide. Certification for ministry encourages us in another direction. Perhaps we need to introduce a Hindu religious
distinction here. In Hinduism, there is the pujari, the trained worship leader who knows the scriptures by heart, the chants and
prayers, the rubrics about when to light fires, swing incense, toss

flowers, and sprinkle water. This job belongs to a well-trained caste that has to study for years. When worship is needed, prayers to be said, the pujari is called on. However, this person is not expected to be holy or wise.

The sanyasi is a holy person who has renounced everything and spends the day in meditation and silence, depending on poor meals from begging or work in a little garden, with maybe the sky for a roof and the earth for a bed. That is the person who is not only sought out as holy but as wise. Sanyasis are asked about all kinds of things that a family counselor or therapist might be asked about in the West. They are not experts on anything necessarily academic although some are very academic indeed. They certainly do not lead the worship or preach as such. In India when a Christian minister was reported for trying to illegally convert Hindus to Christianity, the police showed up at the Christian ashram where the minister led a life of quiet prayer. "Oh," said the police, "there is a mistake. You are not a missionary, you are a holy man."

Dialogue can take place in quiet places. Taizé is a little village in eastern France. To get there from Paris, one must take a train, change to a bus, and then get off and walk up a steep hill. The food is terrible, hot water available in theory only, barracks and bunks are the luxuries for the older visitors. The community was started by Protestant monks, a dozen or so, who prayed together three times a day and offered hospitality. Now it is a community that includes Roman Catholics and tens of thousands of young people come every year to an impossible week of faith sharing, meditative singing, and nothing close to what passes for entertaining youth ministry. The charism for dialogue and hospitality comes out of an initial openness to prayer and quiet.

Years ago, I persuaded my colleagues in campus ministry to get some Taizé brothers living in New York to come down to South Carolina for a retreat weekend. It looked like a disaster in the making. Eighty college students, mostly mainstream Protestants and a few Catholics, sat on the floor around two brothers. One was Swedish and a Lutheran, the other an American Catholic. Neither brother maintained eye contact, both seemed to mumble unintelligibly, and then, the young people popped up, broke into groups, and did the faith sharing the brothers asked them to do. Later, they sang beautifully short Latin songs (Latin being nobody's language, the music was written by a Protestant), and prayed around the cross brought from France. This continued for a night and a day. The brothers violated all the rules for public speaking and youth ministry. But no learned skills can do better than the gratuitous ability we call a charism and they have the charism and they have it because they are dedicated to prayer, silence, and listening.

Perhaps it is the overly verbal Christian worship that has contributed to the shadow that has replaced dialogue. We do not have a tradition of the nonverbal and the verbal blocks the spiritual realities that are protected by silence and accessed by listening. A scholar I met went to India for a Christian-Hindu-Buddhist dialogue. I asked if he meditated, but he said only from time to time. I asked if any monks came to the scholarly meeting. He said yes. What did they contribute? The scholars asked them to make a presentation. When their time came, the monks processed in wearing their robes, sat down, and each presented an object to the assembly: a rock, a flower, and a bowl of water. They sat in front of the objects for thirty minutes of silence, got up, bowed, and left. This seemed delightful to me, but the scholar was in despair—no paper, no research, no footnotes, nothing to talk about! Nothing to talk about except the mystery of reality.

The core of the reality under the shadow of angry ideology is compassion and peace. As part of its foundation Judaism celebrates the forgiveness of Joseph who could have wrecked vengeance on his brothers who had thought of killing him before selling him into slavery. Before Joseph stand virtually the twelve tribes of Israel represented by the brothers who are confronted by compassion and reconciliation. For Christians this is Jesus at the resurrection saying, "Shalom!" to the men who deserted him. Nothing can be crueler than the isolation of betrayal and abandonment and Jesus suffered that. If anyone had rights to blast away, he on Easter day most certainly did. But he does not. In Catholic Church liturgies, we do—verbally—try to reproduce this by praying for peace and extending the kiss of peace to all around us before receiving the Eucharist. We also pray, "Forgive us our trespasses as we forgive those who trespass against us." Some people walk out at this time, maybe just after swiping past and "getting" Communion. So much for communion and compassion.

However, there is another scene we could look at. See Abraham and Josette in the cemetery in Poland where Abraham's mother was buried before the Nazi invasion and the death camps. The stones are overturned and the ground weedy. Josette walks and walks in circles trying to find the grave. "Abraham," she asks, "don't you care where your mother is buried." He, sitting in the middle of the cemetery, says, "She knows we're here." This is the hope of someone others would call a secularized Jew. That label is an ideological one. The reality here is a listener whose outrageous sufferings did not cancel his humanity and who waits under the silent sky knowing that the dead know that we love them. From such hope comes dialogue.

Chapter 5

Nothing Personal:
Lawyers and Ministry
As Business

A small incident from my past has become emblematic of a crisis that blew up thirty years later in the Catholic Church in the United States. I was applying to the Catholic School Department in a small diocese and parked my car by the Cathedral School. When I came out I saw some Cathedral students from an upper story splatter my old Volkswagen with lacquer. The estimated repair was $200, which in those days represented half a month's salary. When I presented the claim to the insurance agency representing the diocese I was only offered half. I was naïve enough to be astonished. I was a teacher in the diocese, earning $400 a month. I needed to make two months' deposit to get an apartment, and now the diocese was going to make me pay a quarter of my month's wages to fix something they were responsible for. I said no to the offer not knowing what to do next. A week later, I returned because it was an offer better than nothing and taking one's employer to small claims court could lead to real problems. Then I was really astonished. The agent said the offer was no longer an option. I would have to sue to get the money. Later, I met the chancellor, a young priest, and I told him the story. He was very sympathetic, but nothing ever got done about it.

Now thirty years later, a commission of lay people have lacerated American bishops in their study of the sex abuse scandals and the additional scandal of how too many bishops have dealt with it. Specifically, the bishops were taken to task for playing hardball with the victims following the advice of insurance companies and lawyers. Many bishops could not be accused of being pastors in the face of the crisis, but more like CEOs. Would this be new behavior or typical behavior of many bishops not only in the face of sex abuse but of many other pastoral challenges? At any rate, the commission called for more pastors and fewer administrators in the episcopacy.

As a priest at graduate school, I used to search out the law students in the dining room and sit with them. After all, in the Gospels, Jesus goes after the lawyers and the priests as much as anyone. The lawyers were not amused at my preference for their company.

As a priest, I know very well why Jesus targeted both priests and lawyers. When I was an administrator, some community members came to me to ask that our summer religion camp be made independent, that is, forced to get its own insurance and tax-exempt status. Summer camps were potentially accidents and lawsuits waiting to happen. I did not force the separation. We were in home mission territory, Catholics were less than 3 percent of the population, the camp was part of our religious formation program in a four-county area with only one small Catholic school. The whole enterprise of religious community, school, and parishes had been an enormous risk. Why not continue? I have never known the Gospel to be served without risk.

In fact, this community of Roman Catholic Oratorians in South Carolina had founded the first integrated Southern Catholic School in 1954. This took enormous courage. Lawyers would have advised against it. In fact, most of the laws of South Carolina at the time were against it. Many parishioners who otherwise would have made use of the school declined and not all of them for racist reasons. Some were simply afraid of the risk. I came into this situation just ten years later when the public swimming facilities of the whole state had been shut down rather than integrate. Now when I hear of "legal" reasons for this or that policy, I am not impressed. The law could not be a motivating force then and does not make much of an impression on me now. When the Gospel mandates something, and we have not gotten around to all the mandates of the Bible, then I believe action is required. But when a lawyer comes at me, I have a hard time being patient. If the law as I knew it had better served justice, I might be more sympathetic. If the Gospel were better-served by law, I would be very happy.

Racism is not all that kept segregation going, but also the power of the law. Conventional Christians do not violate the law. Bad people are in jail and good people are not. This so dominates ordinary consciousness that children automatically pick it up. A group of seventh graders looking at drawings of jails, prisoners, and guards in the Book of Acts were asked who the prisoners were. They responded, of course, bad people. The shock of the Book of Acts comes when we see the good people being arrested and imprisoned. It is part of the Christian heritage. The American civil rights movement was a restoration of something lost in tradition.

This is not to say that coercion, the force of the law, does not have a place. Some people will never do right unless there is a penalty for doing wrong. Perhaps many people are in that category. Certainly authority, even in the church, must sometimes rely on penalties. Perhaps even a bishop in the day-to-day operations of a diocese must impose penalties from time to time. But my overall sense is that lawyers, law, and penalties are overused. This does not mean that we should always blame lawyers. Sometimes, church personnel use penalties that are outside of both the Gospel and the law. Such penalties represent the rule of persons rather than law and that is worse. The authority of Catholic bishops came up once in a serious discussion I was having with colleagues. I wanted to make the case, in front of Protestants, that the Gospel and canon law restricted the bishop. Other Catholics there thought this was a joke. In practice, bishops could do what they wanted barring a huge barrage of publicity to the contrary. This is cynical capitulation but I do not believe that it is restricted to Catholicism, but it was again a major point in the lay commission report to American Catholic bishops. The commission pointed out that too many bishops had ignored the rules that require advise and consent of bodies they must operate with in extraordinary administration. A good canon lawyer, and a brave one at that, would have been helpful.

I was asked once if church administration was loving and supportive. Where did its ministers get love and support? Unfortunately, love and support translate into responsibility and responsibility is now more a legal term defined by courts than it is a moral reality energized by faith. One example that is very bloody at the moment is the swing the Catholic Church has made against the priests accused of sex abuse. They have gone from being coddled to being grilled. Because housing, work, and identity are all tied up for the typical Roman Catholic priest, the "temporary" administrative suspension that takes place at the time of the accusation is something similar to a divorce, a job loss, or an eviction. Although the new guidelines go into great detail about all aspects of the process following the accusation there is only one line for the falsely accused: every effort will be made to restore the priest's reputation. Period. No procedures or guidelines are in place to measure how successfully this policy was followed. You can imagine that if such brevity had been used for the accusers the policy would be pointless. Since anyone talking with the accused can be involved in the trials, the priest is isolated in many dioceses and anyone approaching him is vulnerable as a potential witness. The strength of Catholicism evaporates in the face of such an onslaught. Zen or radical Protestantism would be more helpful to the falsely accused Catholic priest than what little a diocese provides.

Perhaps the church administrators mean that its ministers should rely on God for their support and not on church structures or programs. The mention of God in many administrative meetings of the church is not common. Prudence is a virtue and it dictates that ordinary means should be used to ensure the proper use of church assets. Here we bring on the lawyers and insurance people again. If we want to see their impact, we could attend certain parochial school workshops that are often given around the theme that the schools must be operated similar to businesses; and many are. The most notorious example is from Catholic higher education. In some cases, Catholic universities and colleges survive on the practice borrowed from secular schools of using "adjunct" faculty who, if they worked full time (illegal, but not unheard of), would earn less than $20,000 a year. The market glutted by teachers makes this possible. Who said that the market was the parameter of social justice? Some church-affiliated schools still do two radical things: open the doors to the poor unconditionally and rely on providence to provide. Relying on providence is not a business plan but most Catholic schools were founded for the poor and depended on providence. Something along the way redefined the parochial school as a business. Perhaps there would be less of a quarrel with this if the business of the school were truer to its mission as a church enterprise. The consistent exclusion of those needing scholarships has led to becoming less Catholic both in practice and in spirit. The exclusion of the poor usually results in a school that has only a minority of Catholics. If some sort of evangelization took place among the nonbelievers and something explicitly ecumenical took place among the nonbelievers, it would be worthwhile. But usually a very watery "nondenominational" approach results in what is basically a secular or civil religious option.

As long as church missions are defined by accountants, lawyers, and insurance people, we will have only a shadow of a church ministry. Such domination of these professions would have wiped out the early church where persecution did not. It has resulted in very ambiguous practices that, in the Roman Catholic Church at least, failed to meet a terrible crisis. The lay commission reported to the bishop that the actual problem was more than ambiguity. The problem was the lack of ethics. A recent and powerful book about Christian ethics and business discusses managing "as if faith mattered" (Alford and Naughton, 2001). It is written to help secular society live by the principles of Catholic social justice in the business world. The church that teaches social justice as a cure for the sins of secular society should know that physicians should heal themselves first.

Chapter 6

Evading Focus, Losing God, or, What Was the Question?

A nun I knew worked a heavy schedule as a rural nurse among the poor in Appalachia. Every imaginable demand was made on her. Part of her identity and mission was a deep sense of God so she decided to make a special kind of retreat. *Poustinia* is a Russian word for a hermitage and she chose a place that provided the *Poustinia* style retreat. It included the hermitage, simple food, and the Bible. That was it. No tape players, no radio, nothing but silence. Nothing to read except the Bible. She thought this was a wonderful contrast to her daily existence when she made the arrangements, but as the day drew near, so did the dread of the retreat. Finally, in a kind of a fog she arrived at the first day of the retreat. On stepping inside the hermitage, she heard an inner voice say, "Am I not good enough company for you?" In the Hindu scriptures we can find this very challenging description of the basis of ministry:

> In the center of the castle of Brahmin [God], our own body, there is a small shrine in the form of a lotus-flower, and within can be found a small space. We should find who dwells there, and we should want to know the One. . . . The little space within the heart is as great as this vast universe. The heavens and earth are there, and the sun, and the moon, and the stars; fire and lightening and winds are there; and all that now is and all that is not; for the whole universe is in the

One and the One dwells within our heart. (Chandogya Upanishad 8)

Questioning whether or not God is good enough company for us is surely a shadow over ministry. Other religions that take God as good company find our Western hearts dried out. Another priest I knew had given lots of workshops along the lines of theological and pastoral updating, but he was asked to give a retreat to priests and he was very reluctant. He went to an old priest who had decades of experience and asked advice. "Get them to pray!" said the veteran. When I was writing about teaching prayer in the 1970s, spirituality was a hard sell among priests or Protestant colleagues in campus ministry. Once, upon coming home with two colleagues, one Methodist, one Presbyterian, I was asked about my prayer life. My friends and I bonded over social justice issues and they had never had a peer who was committed to such work and "piety." I felt a bit like a native of somewhere with an anthropologist sticking a microphone in my face. I tried to explain meditation, psalms for morning and evening prayer, and the daily Eucharist. When I finished, my Methodist friend puffed on his pipe and said, "I've often thought I should have a devotional life." Later, when I was in John Wesley's London house, a shrine of Methodism, I sent my friend a postcard of the little room Wesley used in the morning and in the evening for private prayer. The Methodists certainly started out with a method for the spiritual life. Now, if anyone wants an excuse not to pray, ministry is as good as it gets. Everything we do we do for God. The work is never done so there is not time for prayer. If we are praying and someone needs us, we go from God to God. So there. We find God everywhere except in our own hearts.

What has been said about dialogue coming from silence and ministry resisting business models is really a God question. Certainly if all the prudent structures regarded as necessary today result in a secularized staff interchangeable with any skilled social worker or counselor, then the ministry is over. God is not an extra. Pious people without skills have done damage, and secular people with skills have helped, but this does not abolish God because it does not abolish the ultimate questions about meaning. Frankly, without God all were are doing is making people comfortable on death row. Eventually they and us will be swallowed up by a void. A society without God was once unthinkable except by the most radical people who could live with despair. Now God can go and despair is kept at bay by the most inauthentic means possible: modern variations on bread and circuses—shopping malls and sports TV.

The hermitage retreat was the very polar end of bread and circuses. This was a meeting with God, not time wasted or spent with friends or work or vacation. In my own life, I probably did not make such a retreat until a few years after ordination. I had been on community retreats with a preacher taking us through various topics, hit and miss, but nothing so beautiful and so stark as the hermitage. The first real retreat came when I had a chance to go on what was then rather new, a directed retreat. Instead of a general conference, the retreatant meets with the director once a day and is then given some scripture to pray over for twenty-four hours. Other than Eucharist, there are no other common gatherings except for silent meals. It lasted nine days.

I was in the mountains of North Carolina, far from work and my fellow priests. In fact, none of the other priests who registered showed up for the retreat. So I was there with nineteen Roman Catholic nuns. My retreat director was a woman I did not know. I asked for the only priest on the team but I did not have seniority and was bumped on that choice. My other choice, a well-known nun, canceled due to the death of her mother. So a nun I did not know or particularly want was my director for nine days.

The retreat house had burned down some months before so we met in a motel reserved for us. We walked up a steep hill to the rectory and church for mass, meals, and private conferences. Because we were Roman Catholics scattered all over the Southeast, we asked if we could talk during meals so we could get to know one another better. This was granted. We also had two impromptu parties to celebrate birthdays, but otherwise we were good and observant retreatants!

Proof that this was going to be another kind of retreat came the first minute of the conference. Sister asked how God and I were doing. Not how the community and I were doing, not how was the bishop or church and I doing, or parish and I, or anything else but God. I had never been asked that question before. I noticed a box of tissues next to me and wondered what they were for. In five days, I found out. The flood of tears came when I had to deal with the suffering that permeated much of my life. I discovered that my preference for quiet prayer was, in my heart . . . not my head, a preference for staying out of the way so God would not notice me and have me crucified some more. Could I surrender to God? Could I trust Him? I thought I did already because I preached that and certainly my head said that I believed it. But not my guts.

> Father,
> I abandon myself into your hands;
> do with me what you will.
> Whatever you may do, I thank you:
> I am ready for all, I accept all.
> Let only your will be done in me,
> and in all your creatures -
> I wish no more than this, O Lord.
>
> Into your hands I commend my soul:
> I offer it to you with all the love of my heart,
> for I love you, Lord, and so need to give myself,
> to surrender myself into your hands without reserve,
> and with boundless confidence,
> for you are my Father.
>
> Charles deFoucauld

It took two years to say this prayer. My guts said that if I prayed it, I would be tested by God with cancer and my best friend would die! Now the guts never said this in a loud voice or in a distinctive way, but there back in the shadows it was very insistent that surrendering would be devastating. After all, I had not surrendered yet and lots had been taken already. Where would the rest go if I let go?

Letting go was the best thing that ever happened to me. Active ministers can take comfort in knowing that surrendering to God has the practical effect of infusing more energy and creativity in pastoral work. A certain pragmatism in mysticism gets over-looked. John of the Cross teaches that more gets done the more time spent in prayer. After we surrender to God, prayer does not seem an option anymore. Our active lives seem now to depend on it. This does not mean that most in ministry will be in danger of running off to the cloister, a fear that seems to keep many away from prayer and tied to some unbelievable burdens, mostly in ad-ministration. But if the majority will not run to the cloister it does explain why a growing minority seek more silence and meditation though too often they think they must abandon busy Christianity to find a still point in their lives.

In Roman Catholic circles, the best way to kill off a spiritual practice is to label it "monastic." Monasticism is a very conserva-tive and conserving life choice. What some still label monastic is, as a matter of fact, something that was common to all Christians but got lost except in the cloister. We need not be cloistered to learn to stop morning and evening for prayer or to read the Bible as prayer, but we must go to the cloister to find a teacher. We need not imitate monks but we must transform the common Christian spiri-tual practices and make them part of our lives. The alternative is overwork, TV, the shopping mall, or the asceticism of the runner or weight room.

The foreign mission experience might teach us something. Mis-sionaries with an activist Christianity arrive in cultures where the non-Christian tradition is to pray morning, noon, and evening, per-haps spending time in meditative chanting or silence.

The missionaries teach a form of Christianity that reserves these practices to monks and cloistered nuns. The converts lose a source of soul making that was valued by their culture but cut off by Western activist Christians. Perhaps Christians should go to countries where the general population still prays in the morning and evening. Gandhi was certainly no quietist. He led the libera-tion of India from an ashram, a house of prayer. He observed a day of silence each week and would not depart from that even in a crisis that required him to write notes. This might seem odd to us since he was communicating, but there is something spiritual about not hearing our own voices for twenty-four hours. Central to the ashram life with Gandhi was morning and evening prayer; roll was taken at each. Morning prayer was especially hard because he insisted that they pray at 4:00, the hour the poor did before work. More privileged Hindus prayed later, but Gandhi was not interested in that. His assassination took place as he went to evening prayer. The assassin knew he was faithful to this schedule and knew where to find him. Gandhi's last words were a prayer, "Eh, Ram!" This is miserably translated in English as "Oh, God!" and in our profane society can be taken as a cheap exclamation of horror. It was not such an expression in his life. God was the goal of his life and all that he did flowed from the unifying experience of this search for God.

The American civil rights movement took its initial energy from the African-American experience of church. God here is not a left-brain experience. The services are long and nobody seems to mind. An "amen" in a church of Christians willing to suffer for civil rights is another kind of surrender to God. If I were afraid of surrendering to God because of my fear of the cross, imagine a church surrendering to God to be able to embark on civil rights. Such a mission inevitably is bound to the cross. It also requires prayer and abandonment to God and never relinquishing the vision that is, after all, a vision given by God and not conjured up by ourselves.

Two great movements of the last century had their home base in prayer. Today new forms are being born to carry ministry and prayer as partners. The ecumenical community of Taizé was previously mentioned. Roman Catholic versions are also available. In Rome, during the turmoil of 1968, three young men in high school gathered every evening for vespers—psalms, scripture, and intercessions. They shared what they thought should be their response considering the concrete challenges of the day. This gathering grew and they were given a rundown, mildewed church, the little San Egidio, where they ran burlap up the wall, across the floor, and up the other wall, and sat on the floor for prayer. Today, the leaders are in their late forties, and the movement of "San Egidio" involves thousands in Rome and elsewhere. They are used and trusted internationally because of their work in developing countries and with immigrants to Italy. Still, the format remains the same: gathering every evening for vespers, now sung with gusto by a huge crowd, and meals together four times a week. From their ministry has sprung up something that touches a good part of the world.

In Paris, a community of monks, nuns, and laity can be found in the middle of the city in the church of St. Gervais just behind City Hall. Although there are more things to do in Paris than pray, several hundred Parisians gather every day for evening prayer and Mass lasting ninety minutes. Shorter services are offered in the morning and at noon. On Sundays, the church is packed. It is known for its beautiful music, biblical preaching, and ecumenical and interfaith work. The order is new and only recently approved after several decades of ministry. Hundreds of monks and nuns and hundreds more of laity are members. Their spirituality is focused on the city as a new desert and to the ecumenical realities of monasticism. The symbol for the core of their life is the city of Jerusalem, the city as metaphor for their lives in France and the real city of Jerusalem. Neither place is easy to live, but both places are modern-day crossroads where a house of prayer and outreach has a powerful presence.

In the United States, awareness has grown in the church and in the synagogue that the rejected God of our childhood needs to be replaced by a living God that meets the prophets and saints in the real world. This God still keeps bushes burning to humble us. This God's stillness is the silent language of love. We can thank all kinds of Christian and Jewish writers who dared to reintroduce themselves to the God of saints and prophets and then shared that experience with us. Words such as prayer, mysticism, contemplation, and even monasticism are no longer impolite but are living realities being explored again.

The value of this recovery to ecumenism cannot be underestimated. We seem to be heading into another era of division over moral practice just as we recover a common sense of sacraments and church order. But nothing can keep us from sitting in silence together and on a regular basis. My own tradition within the Oratory of St. Philip Neri is exactly that gift. The parish was founded in 1575 when a Latin liturgy separated the laity from the Church's prayer. Part of the solution was a kind of Methodist cottage meeting in the afternoon with faith sharing and talks and singing. In the evening they gathered for quiet prayer. Today, our prayer is not really just for the community but for the public and it consists of a fair amount of silence together and the door is open to anyone seeking God. Sitting together in silence and anchoring this kind of prayer every day with the door open and inviting is, in fact, our chief ministry, our reason to exist. Some years ago a very zealous and prayerful nun came to join us in ministry. She could spend a good deal of time in private prayer but she could not understand why we would rush back to the house just to sit in silence. If we remember that silence is not punitive, but the language of love then the central experience of God can be shared in that silent gathering together of an otherwise divided or busy family.

The spiritual realities of compassion, silence, presence, and awe can be explored and even experienced together in silence. Newman, one of the world's great preachers, nevertheless thought that verbalizations were a loss and that the more reticence the more room for God. Everyone's ministry could be summed up by saying that we work with others to make room for God.

Chapter 7

Who Is in Charge Here?

Priests are not often prophets. In fact, in scripture, they fall into two different categories. But priests have been prophetic and they were so in South Carolina in 1956. The integration of the school that was accomplished by Oratorian priests in Rock Hill was not only a matter of taking on lawyers and the civic community but also their fellow Catholics in the parishes they served. The founding of the school was at the time of the Supreme Court decision that separate schools for the races could not by definition be equal and therefore should be abolished. However, the integration of the school had come a few years before the Supreme Court decision and it was done strictly for religious reasons. It was the decision of the priests, not a parish council or a consultation of the laity. The decision was made as a moral one with no possible alternatives except sinful ones.

Now was this dictatorship? Patriarchy? It certainly was not democratic. If it had been left up to the people it would not have been done. Integration happened not only against the wishes of lawyers and other prudent advisors, but against the wishes of a large number of parents whose children were, after all, at risk. Protests and demonstrations were held, and crosses were burned. But the school went ahead with a lay faculty of women volunteers from Boston and a local woman as principal. It was done quietly. An inquiry was made about a national news program contrasting "Little Rock" (Arkansas), the scene of integration carried out by soldiers protecting the black students and "Rock Hill" where integration had occurred, in contrast, more peacefully. The Oratorians refused coverage, sure that publicity would really put the school at risk. This lonely task had no real support from the bishop (but no opposition either). It was something done in a prophetic way. By definition, it would not have been done any other way.

Within the Catholic and Orthodox tradition is a kind of leadership that can be and was arbitrary and patriarchal. The essence of the tradition was a listening leadership that discerned with the community and sometimes sided with a minority of the community. Minorities can be right and certainly must be protected and this tradition of leadership has the advantage of the prophetic edge if the spirit is allowed to operate.

Now Americans are nearly automatically opposed to this although our constitution says that the president be elected directly and so we have had presidents who won a plurality of votes that were unevenly distributed and so lost in the electoral college. This system has never been corrected because the smaller states benefit from it.

Americans otherwise prefer majority rule and this shows up in ministry. More than one workshop facilitator has started out training new councils and boards by reminding them that "None of us is as smart as all of us!" But this is not true. Group decisions unless strictly governed by certain rules will result in something less intelligent than some members of the group. Years ago, a popular psychology magazine published a simulation game from NASA. The premise was that the team was stranded on the moon. Dozens of objects could be selected for the successful escape and each individual made a prioritized list. The lists were shared and a group list emerged. If the rules were followed then the group list was always objectively better than any one list. The rules were strict: no bargaining, no compromises, and each person's reason had to be listened to and objections stated and agreed upon. Once when I ran the game, I knew the parish well and put two very aggressive people in the same group. I was pretty sure the individuals in that group would score higher because they would be outtalked by the two aggressors who would find it hard to follow the rules. That was certainly the result. They were the only group out of eight that had the problem.

Today, the lowest common denominator more often rules rather than wise discernment. Communities that elected abbots and abbesses who would listen to everyone, senior and junior, and make decisions are now mostly reduced to some kind of democratic vote if not an actual free-for-all. No wonder so many Roman Catholic communities have quietly shelved a common purpose in favor of "live and let live." There would be no reason to join such a community, of course. We can all live and let live without the countless meetings and revisions of government and mission statements that plague communities still trying to make decisions that ratify everyone. The mainstream denominations are struggling with this also. What had been Protestant/Catholic splits over doctrine and practice have now become multiple splits within the major churches. Once divided and broken, the church may be brought back together again. When authority is the issue and the majority wish to reserve authority to themselves as individuals, then diversity, a great value, trumps unity and too often unnecessarily. Authority, as Cardinal Newman knew, rests on individual conscience but there does not have to be by nature a split between the two. Our consciences can discover the authority that can speak for the community, living and dead. Admitting the dead as witnesses to authoritative decisions is, according to G.K. Chesterton, real democracy and real inclusion. To assume that the times are so different and that the past must be thrown out rather than developed is an Enlightenment prejudice. In postmodern times when plurality is a value in itself and room is made for all kinds of cultures, then the community tradition should surely hold some place. Of course, this is assuming that someone knows about the tradition and our own self-induced cultural Alzheimer's loss of collective memory had eradicated our own treasures from the past.

The greatest example of the last century when prophetic authority and the community leaders worked together was the ministry of Pope John XXIII. The Second Vatican Council was his prerogative alone to call and call it he did—and he listened to the council. It was made up of appointees of Pius XII, who was accused as either morally inept or an actual Nazi collaborator. That Pius XII would be so regarded now would be a shock to John XXIII, but John also knew that the church was overdue for change. Change needs consensus if it is not to turn into a revolution accomplished by the few. The few trying to create a revolution both from the right and left is another story. But, the Catholic Church making as many changes as possible without schism remains a mystery that has not been fully explained or explored. More pluralism is demanded and not all of it of equal worth. More change could be accomplished if the leadership were true to its own words and to a tradition of radical holiness.

Yet do we the people want holiness? Consider the story of the Catholic priest, one of the few nonreligious-order priests canonized, John Vianney. The women's sodality gave him a stipend for an early weekday mass which they attended fervently as a group. The stipend was given for a "special intention" but nothing else was said as to why the mass was being offered. Finally, after nearly a decade of this, he asked the sodality what the intention was. The president said, "Your transfer." The presence of the holy, integrated person as we know from the prophets and Jesus can threaten the majority.

In the 1970s an American psychologist researching in the Netherlands got results showing our ambiguous relationship to authority and leadership. She managed to get the cloistered contemplative Carmelite nuns to take part in the research. The prioresses and subprioresses came to the university to sit quietly while the electrodes attached to them recorded their ability to reach a meditative state. They also took psychological tests. Consistently, the subprioresses were able to more quickly reach a meditative stage and they also scored as more-integrated personalities on the tests. Now how was that? The office of prioress is an elected office. The subprioress is appointed by the prioress. One explanation is that the more-integrated personalities were not popular with the majority who preferred someone a little weaker. But the prioresses were prudent enough to appoint the more-integrated to be able to get their job done. I was an elected superior and I can say that in my case I believe the fear of the more-integrated person got me elected as a compromise candidate.

The preference for a less demanding leadership spills over into the local church. A kind of conspiracy exists between the pulpit and the pew, between administrations and its ministers. The conspiracy compromises the holy and the prophetic. "Don't rock the boat" helped lead many bishops and their administrations into the mishandling of sex abuse—the worst crisis of the American Catholic Church. It has led to many crises in many different places from other Christian churches to politics and business. The shadow over any ministry with any organization is the fear of the prophet. King David was an exception to the rule when he let Nathan confront him. The usual pattern is Elijah up against Ahab and Jezebel. Parish councils are no fonder of the prophet than the old-style pastor.

So board meetings, council meetings, and committee meetings take the place of authority and holiness, prophecy and spirit. Is this because such meetings are productive? No. Management magazines of big business are the first to say how unproductive meetings are even when they have a specific task to do. What is really operating if the meetings are counterproductive? The attraction of masochism should not be underrated here. It is easy to spot masochism in the self-flagellations and grim fasting in the past, but now instead of wearing hair shirts and whipping ourselves, we go to meetings. Why we go will be clearer to another age that might well see the same hidden love of pain just re-emerging in another kind of organization. In theological terms, meetings can be just another version of salvation through works. The nice thing about the medieval church was the indulgence in which a penitent could substitute certain prayers for doing bigger penances. If our organizations offered indulgences so we could substitute our presence at meetings for say, spending part of the morning praying or going for a swim, would we not prefer the indulgence? Even if such indulgences were sold, would we not buy some from time to time?

Our time is, then, the final issue. The old strict Sabbath was one way to call a halt to dehumanized loss of time. An ecumenist in Jerusalem told me that the Muslim Friday observance, the Jewish Sabbath, and the Christian Sunday gave the city three days of relative peace. Bombs are not the usual danger in our cities, but lack of sleep and overwork are. A humanized sense of unrushed purpose focused on the most important things in our lives remains out of the reach of many. The solution is not long sermons and extended Sunday school, but a recovery of joy and purpose. Nothing cuts into joy and purpose more than enforced wasted time. The fact that we get paid for it is the only thing that makes it tolerable. I sometimes wonder if the ill temper of God pictured in the scriptures came from too many fruitless and repetitive meetings with people who don't follow through.

The following are some suggestions to bring a little light and lightness to our ministry:

1. Stay focused on the mission statement. If we are running all over trying not only to cover the bases but to play basketball and football at the same time, then we need lots of meetings. Competent people focused on their ministry need fewer meetings.
2. Demand more trust and more accountability. These go together. The trustworthy want to be accountable. Agree on the mission and the measurements and get on with it.
3. Do not hold meetings merely to receive reports. Reports are made at meetings because people don't read reports and wait for them to be read aloud. This is a waste. Bring reactions to the reports.
4. Use a spiritual director, counselor, friend, or therapist to process the raw meat of your emotions. Don't expect the group to do this. The group doesn't like it and really can't help. Before the meeting, find out what your particular ax is and grind it outside the group.
5. Pretend you really are stranded on the moon and that proper listening and negotiation is essential to life and death. If the meeting is not about life and death, don't go.
6. Don't go to the meeting to show off. If you must show off find some kids somewhere and entertain them.

These points are offered as a guide to an attitude that could free us from the guilt we feel when we use common sense and skip meetings. Our absence probably will not be noticed. And if we need a really good excuse not to go, we can fall back on the one we use not to pray: we are leaving God at the meeting to meet God in the needs of our neighbor.

Chapter 8

The Family of the Minister:
Sex, Love, and Grief

Vincent de Paul was the great seventeenth-century servant of the poor. He was a realistic but untiring working both in the city and the countryside among the destitute whom he considered to be his masters. One day an impoverished cousin, poorly educated and badly dressed, appeared at the door to his house. He was mortified and made the cousin go to the backdoor. It took him longer to claim the wounded in his own family than it did to accept the needs of strangers.

And so we come to the minister's family. Now this means both married and unmarried clergy. Catholic priests are seen as not having a family because they are not married. Of course, this would mean that priests are hatched and not born into a family. All ministers, married and unmarried, have family and live with the history of that family as part of their ministry. Whether the family was normally dysfunctional, really dysfunctional, or exceptional in their happiness, must be worked through.

I had been ordained about a year when a young mother came to talk to me. She had problems dealing with her own parents. But the problem was her mother's goodness! The woman did not know how to live with the fact that she could not remember her mother making a false move or failing in any way. Her mother was a positive role model and the burden was too much.

After this episode, I realized that everyone's first problem is that they have parents. Parents can be good or less than good, but they are problems in any case because they are parents. Children at any age are problematic because they are after all children. It does not matter if they are successful in society or not, they are still children. As they grow up, matters only become more problematic because they fall in love and get married. Children having their own spouses and possibly children of their own can create anxieties if not problems outright. Marital problems, especially divorces, are never between a couple alone. The others suffering loss are any surviving parents and, often enough, other siblings. With no end of caring, there is no end of anxieties. That is both the good news and the bad news.

The minister with parents is a minister at work, examining personal challenges and blessings. They often speak enough like their parents, not only to their own children, but to those they minister. The parents are the "invisible" partners in the ministry. Sometimes the parents are the invisible partners the minister is still reacting to. So these ministers sound similar to their parents, but in reverse. In both cases, the parents are still dominating.

When we listen to ourselves and others, we need to listen deeply to hear who is really speaking. Naturally, the same applies when listening to authority or evading authority. The shadow of our family history intrudes because most of our actions, even our "helpful" ones, at least start out as power moves and we learn about power in the middle of a family. As we learn to minister less from power or at least learn to be aware of how we use power, we become freer and more responsible for our own actions.

A first step for many toward this sense of freedom and responsibility is to give up the false responsibility for family wounds in childhood. Many children think that what they do, even in secret, "causes" things to happen. At the same time, they are not likely to take public responsibility or talk about it. Whatever they think they caused is carried around as a private burden. Most trained ministers know this, but the kind of self-knowledge necessary to see it in ourselves usually takes a spiritual partner or director and time alone from time to time. Information provided by specialists in dysfunctional families can be misleading here. Everyone in a dysfunctional family has a role to play, but when it is the children born into the dysfunctional situation, they are hardly responsible even though later on they can feel guilty in the knowledge of the role they had in keeping family pain going. God is more merciful than many family specialists whose ability to label people is better than their ability to affirm and heal. The academic grounding of these specialists may be quite sound, but academics forget that understanding by itself can lead to paralysis. After all, Hamlet was a university student. Certainly the child within will not become the adult within without affirmation and healing. What child with such adult models would want to become an adult?

Grieving over family history, especially when faced with social pressures, can grow worse in middle-aged ministers who are "successful" and facing a congregation of families with portfolios, lawyers, and trust funds. Such a congregation is ultrasensitive to family history because members reflexively protest their own assets by directing their children to other families with the same assets. Those assets are not likely to be found in dysfunctional families, or so they think. In practice, old- and new-money families are as riddled with alcoholism, drugs, infidelity, and desertion as most other segments of society. Why everyone keeps pretending that money, prestige, and power brings not only happiness but morality, I do not know. What the press considers scandals are the norm in life. What would be news is a happy, integrated family whose place in society comes from high principles and not the perpetual making of insider deals or inherited or married wealth.

Actually, coming from a dysfunctional family should make the minister sensitive to what is really going on among the people in any situation. A normal family background could be too rare a thing to help ministers understand in their guts what is really playing out in their mission. In any case, it is my contention that the initial problem is having a family and everyone starts out with that as both an advantage and a disadvantage.

What is harder to get at are the experiences in which everything in the family was proper enough to provide shelter, food, education, and a certain social standing, yet the relationships were distant and cold. Someone coming out of such a situation did not experience communication as communion but as something that happens in formal and appointed times or does not happen at all. One man explained to me that his father died unexpectedly, and that he had never taken the time to take his dad out to lunch so he could tell him that he loved him. A spontaneous hug or acclamation of love could not happen; there had to be an appointment and a restaurant first. Ministering from this experience can make us good executives, but poor lovers and poor pastors. Sometimes late in life, these ministers do find love and the disruption to ministry is severe, but better for them to be loved and love than to continue in what was essentially an icy ministry disguised as efficiency and ability.

As complex as the family is, reducing the family to just the two spouses uncovers how many woman-man relationships get played out in ministry based on the family. The place of women is still ambiguous even in churches, which by policy, allow for women's ordination. I think something more is going on here than just male power plays. Men find something fearful in women. If anyone is from Mars, it may be the woman if inspired fear is the measurement of warrior. An education for most ministers has been provided by their staff who are usually nearly all women. The minister moves between female co-workers and usually a male-dominated administration even in liberal institutions. The minister soon learns that these are two different worlds. In my experience, female co-workers are more honest and perceptive as well as more nurturing. All male administrations are usually still playing out sibling rivalries and who daddy likes best. The realism provided by the women in the local setting counteracts the never-never land of general administration that often bounces between the dry bones of business decisions to thinly disguised competition for the biggest whatever. A minister, woman or man, who has trouble with women will be deprived of a good deal of humanity and therefore, grace. A totally male world will certainly cave in to poor administration, the very thing it believes it is good at. Without the honesty, perception, and nurturing that takes place in the local world of female staff, business suffers.

If men and women are still struggling for real relationships in ministry, then the gay and lesbian community will have a long wait before dialogue is even established. At the present time, gays in ministry are pawns in a power struggle between different factions of the churches. In Roman Catholic circles, liberals try to frighten the Vatican into abolishing celibacy by insisting that too many gays are attracted to the shield provided by compulsory celibacy. They will go so far as to insist that gays cannot minister to the needs of heterosexuals and so their ministry is impaired. The other side insists that gays cannot be priests because their celibacy is worthless as a gift since all they are doing is abstaining from sin. So it is not just conservative-oriented people who are opposed to gays in ministry. The side in favor of inclusion is not necessarily liberal or conservative. They simply insist that all things being otherwise equal, if celibacy is observed, then the issue is not that important. The issue of celibacy is primarily a focal point of Roman Catholicism, but celibacy for gays and lesbians is not just a Roman point of contention. Moreover the gay community is quite diverse and includes people who do not seem to know, as with a number of bishops, that sexual contact with anyone younger than eighteen is a crime. The late activist and writer Paul Monette described in a memoir his affair with a prep school student when he was a teacher. Today, that affair could have gotten him jail time. The explosive issue of adult sexuality touches on youth all the time. The adult community has failed terribly here to be consistently responsible.

Granted all this, and that is a large concession, the real concerns of people opposed and in favor of different kinds of inclusion of gays and lesbians have been displaced by the one side shutting doors and by the other side assuming that the struggle can only be understood as a civil rights matter. Sexuality is far more powerful and primitive than anything else we must deal with. Sexual arousal is not a cognitive function. To sit around and pretend that it is not deeply emotional and disruptive is to think that we are angels with disembodied intellects. (So we were cursed by Descartes and the Enlightenment.) Yet the problem is also intellectual. In Roman Catholic moral theology, the definition of natural law allows for rape and incest to be classified as "natural" sins because they involve a male and female while masturbation and artificial birth control would be classified as "unnatural" since a partner is missing in the one and there is a physical interference with conception in the other. This side of the intellectual argument is seeking to find a way to say that persons and what used to be called natural law is something to be paid attention to without reducing sexuality to mechanics. The other side defines the issues in an existential and isolated way so that persons are detached from both commu-

nal and physical definitions. Some of the dialogue recently emerged
and one source will very likely be Pope John Paul II's contribution
to understanding the nature of the person. But right now the Vatican is a poor sender and the media is a receiver so that resource is
not very accessible. In fact, actual legal and social practice jumps
faster than most of us can react in a human and dialogical way.

Perhaps we can get to a better place for dialogue by remembering that we started by saying that the shadow side of ministry was
the human side. What this century has inherited from the last is a
searing reminder of how destructive human beings can be. We
hardly know what a person is now because so much of the last century was a violation of the person. Our ministry takes place amidst
the reminders of that violence and the human capacity for violence. A certain kind of ministry simply wants to evade such issues
in favor of an optimism that relies on professional standards when
we know that professional standards do not always keep professionals true. A simple kind of ministry relies on goodwill and convention even though we know that goodwill and convention have
failed. The shadow side of ministry is our human selves. Our
common need for the light that enlightens everyone is perennial.

Appendix

Resources for the Shadow Side of Ministry

The emphasis of this book has been on personal experiences. Letting practice and experience dominate is only one method. Behind the practical, resources such as the following also try to capture whole what we experience in parts, fits, and stops, sometimes going in circles, sometimes moving ahead. Reflecting on these resources should help the dialogue that this book is meant to contribute to. Movies, poems, novels, theoretical models, essays, memoirs, and expositions are all available. The human experience of the shadow is the standard material of artists and thinkers. Our market-dominated society does not sell the insights that could make us more reflective and less competitive. But for ministry, they are springs of water coming out of the rocky desert of commercialism.

Stages of Growth or The Stations of the Cross?

At a time when *Lord of the Rings* (Tolkien, 1954/2005) dominates even the popular imagination, need we cite anything more than that? The author, J. R. R. Tolkien, was a devout Roman Catholic who eschewed allegory (in the mode of C. S. Lewis's *The Chronicles of Narnia,* 1950/2000), but nevertheless possessed a deeply Catholic imagination. The symbolic journey of sacrificial love, the common effort it takes even at the end to destroy the ring, biblical images such as bread on the desert journey and water from the rock, dominate in a profoundly religious way a story that does not describe a religion so much as the effects of a faith that is communal and sacramental.

An overlooked classic but well worth dipping into is *The Pilgrim's Progress* (Bunyan, 1684/1966). It was required reading during senior summer reading at the prep school I attended and it was easy to dislike, but the effect and images in the book are classics and emerge constantly from memory and light up daily experiences.

More compact is Georges Bernanos's (1937), *Diary of a Country Priest*. This is the quintessential example of the shadow side of ministry. Robert Bresson made this into a movie that would be a very good resource for ministry training regardless of denomination. Robert Coles used it at Harvard to challenge the imagination of the elite.

A Feast Day Funeral

In *Darkness Visible: A Memoir of Madness*, William Styron (1990/ 1992) uses all his skill to describe his experience with clinical depression. His novel, *Sophie's Choice* (1979/1992), is the insider's view of depression and suicide.

Gertrude von le Fort's (1954) novella *The Song of the Scaffold* was turned into an extraordinary modern opera, *Dialogues of the Carmelites*, by Francis Poulenc, composer, and Georges Bernanos, writer, who had previously adapted it as a play. The Carmelites are the nuns executed near the very end of the reign of terror in the French Revolution. The story's tension centers on the desire of one of the nuns excluded from martyrdom and another who is frightened and leaves only to freely join the nuns on the scaffold. The nuns were free to disperse but stayed together knowing that it would be considered treason and they would be executed. They died singing.

Rod and Staff: Co-Workers

Jean Vanier, a French Canadian, is the founder of L'Arche, the ultimate example of the meshing of mission, staff, and community. It began in France as one community of the mentally disabled and helpers. The community did not help the disabled, but rather lived and worked with them as comembers. The community is still mostly laity and no vows are involved. Many do make a lifetime commitment. Vanier's book *Community and Growth* (1989) is a compendium of years of experience in this ministry. Today L'Arche is an ecumenical and interfaith union of communities scattered around the world.

Helen Alford and Michael Naughton's (2001) *Managing As if Faith Mattered, Christian Social Principles in the Modern Organization* has two introductions by businessmen who are witnesses to the viability of business partnered with ethics. If businesses can operate with respect for their workers and customers, the church could also. This very creative and engaging work challenges the church to implement its own social teachings within its own structures.

The Death of Dialogue

Martin Buber's (1923/1971) *I and Thou* and Reuel Howe's (1963) *Miracle of Dialogue* deserve a reread in these less-than dialogical times. Buber's dense existential German/Hebrew thinking is perhaps not as accessible today as when students were better prepared to tackle such things and even make them popular. Howe is watered down or clarified Buber depending on your point of view.

For Roman Catholics and those in dialogue with them, see Pope Paul VI's classic letter *Paths of the Church (Ecclesiam Suam)*. The statements on dialogue have mostly gotten lost, but it remains the touchstone for those not weary of the culture wars and willing to listen to the other side. In the third section of the papal letter is a detailed evocation of the opportunities and limits of dialogue. Most important to our considerations here is the following:

> If we want to be men's pastors, fathers and teachers, we must also behave as their brothers. Dialogue thrives on friendship, and most especially on service. All this we must remember and strive to put into practice on the example and precept of Christ. (#87, *Ecclesiam Suam*)

Nothing Personal: Lawyers and Ministry As Business

The sobering *Report on the Crisis of the Catholic Church in the United States* was created by a lay commission and presented to the American bishops (2003). After several sections detailing the statistics of abuse, the commission turned to issues of governance. Nearly fifty pages are given to very strong condemnation of a system that is closed-in, dependent more on lawyers than pastoring, and unfaithful even to its own canons.

What was once considered a lurid fiction version of the shadow over church administration can be found in the now relatively tame *True Confessions*. John Gregory Dunne's (1977) novel starts out with a murder that leads to an Archdiocesan benefactor. The cardinal's secretary is supposed to help "take care" of the mess. The novel was also made into a movie starring Robert DeNiro. At the end, DeNiro's character chooses priesthood over ministry as a career and ends up exiled to a desert parish of poor people. On a personal note, at the end of the movie, beaten but whole, DeNiro has the exact look of my first pastor. They could have been brothers and indeed through fiction and film were both purified examples of wounded ministers transformed by the light that finally prevails through the shadows.

Evading Focus: Losing God, or What Was the Question?

The Paulist series of *Classics of Western Spirituality* has an excellent selection of John and Charles Wesley's writings and hymns. I find the affinity between the early Methodists and the early Oratorians under St. Philip Neri in sixteenth-century Rome very heartening.

The Quaker Thomas R. Kelly's *A Testament to Devotion* (1996) is a remarkable book which addresses the spiritual experience that many share across the various divisions in the church.

Kathleen Norris has written among other books *Dakota: A Spiritual Geography* (1993) and *The Cloister Walk* (1996). She is a poet and a Protestant who is a Benedictine oblate. *Dakota* is a discovery of community and the desert tradition in modern America. *The Cloister Walk* is an appreciative dialogue with the impact of monasticism still going despite every effort of different eras to wipe it out.

Teresa of Avila's *Interior Castle* (1979) remains the classic here. She tries to convince her readers of how beautiful they are and that the journey to the center is worth it. Before we invented psychology we had natural experts such as Teresa and John of the Cross. John Welch (1982) has written a clear introduction albeit Jungian to the work of Teresa. His *Spiritual Pilgrim: Carl Jung and Teresa of Avila* works the *Interior Castle* through the process of human individuation.

I hesitate to recommend Thomas Merton's *Contemplative Prayer* (1996), because I found it dense and dry, but a Protestant colleague exhausted by the activism of the 1960s said that the book saved his life. That is high praise and so I pass it on to you who may find it fruitful. Otherwise, Thomas Merton appeals across the board in *Conjectures of a Guilty Bystander* (1966), *Seeds of Contemplation* (1949/1987), *New Seeds of Contemplation* (1962/1972), and the condensation of his journals, *The Intimate Merton: His Life from His Journal,* brilliantly edited by Jonathan Montaldo and Patrick Hart (1999).

The great gift of the Eastern Church is the collection on prayer called the *Philokalia* (1995). A one-volume version is followed by volumes that expand the original material. This compendium of Orthodox spirituality is extremely insightful into both spirituality and psychology.

Concerning the encounter of Christians with other cultures and religions, there is not, I think, a better resource than the work in India of the French priest, Henri LeSaux. An Indian Jesuit told me that LeSaux was only one of two Westerners he believed who had really become Indian. LeSaux took an Indian name, Abhishiktananda (the bliss of the anointed one—the Christ), and published using this identity. He wrote a small book called *Prayer* (1967), which powerfully and succinctly outlines the benefits of living the tensions of two deep spiritualities.

Gandhi's *Letters to the Ashram* (1932) is hard to find, but in these letters back to the Ashram he makes it clear how the search for God, a daily and communal discipline of prayer, and the struggle for Indian freedom were, in his mind, all related.

Donald Lopez is a student of Buddhism and he warns in *Prisoners of Shangri-La: Tibetan Buddhism and the West* (1999) that access to other religions demands an immersion that our cafeteria approach resists.

On the American scene, I recommend the work of the poet Mary Oliver, whose sensibilities communicate the sacred to a modern society, and Wendell Berry's poetry, novels, and essays. Berry is a Kentucky farmer and writer of small books that are critical of the assumptions of secular city folks. His alternative view is beautiful and, dare we say, traditional.

Who Is in Charge Here?

Robert K. Greenleaf's *Servant Leadership: A Journey into the Nature of Legitimate Power and Greatness* (1977) remains at the top of everyone's list on governance. He works on a model of leadership that does not renounce power, but grounds it differently than the blatantly hierarchical models. It does not promote a totally egalitarian model, but something collaborative and ethical.

For evangelicals, Rick Warren's book *The Purpose-Driven Life* (2002) touches on matters of decision making. He is more explicit in *The Purpose-Driven Church* (1995).

Roman Catholic classics go back to *The Rule of St. Benedict.* The *Rule* remains the keystone to understanding the peculiar character of governance by an elected listener and decision maker.

Ignatius Loyola's *Spiritual Exercises* (2000) details another approach to discernment and judgment. Much Ignatian literature is available on the subject, but my impression is that it is rather ignored in practice.

The nineteenth-century classic essay for Roman Catholics is John Henry Newman's (1961) *On Consulting the Faithful in Matters of Doctrine.* Although it got him into some trouble, Newman never abandoned the essay. He derived the principle from his Anglican days studying the early church. He noted that during the early controversies over doctrine it was the bishops who hesitated to develop an orthodox understanding of Jesus while it was the people and their popular religion that decided the matter. Church governance, even in touching doctrine, should involve consulting the faithful. In his Roman Catholic preface to a new edition of an Anglican work, *The Via Media* (1990), Newman outlined the near impossibility of finite church officials ever managing to coordinate properly at one time the traditional three offices of teaching, governance, and worship.

A recent study of different papers presented at a Roman Catholic conference on the present crisis in the American Catholic Church resulted in editors Franklin Oakley and Bruce Russett (2004) publishing *Governance, Accountability, and the Future of the Catholic Church.* For ministers in other traditions, I can only present this material as evidence of the Holy Spirit touching an institution that still needs reform and renewal. Pope John Paul II himself said as much in his letter on ecumenism, *That All May Be One (Ut Unum Sint,* 1995). Here he was bold enough to ask other Christians what the church could do to make its governance more effective and attractive.

The Family of the Minister

The late Polish film director Krzysztof Kieslowski produced a very important series for Polish television called collectively *The Decalogue* (1988). All ten films, nearly an hour each, are in family settings. In his trilogy *The Three Colors: Blue, White, and Red,* I would recommend *Blue* (1993) as a poignant film about the resolution of family issues after the death of a spouse. The film is much more than that, but to know that something religious can acknowledge the shadow side of life and portray plausibly reconciliation and forgiveness is central to the issues that have been raised in this book.

The Brothers Karamazov (1855/1992) is Dostoyevsky's monument to the dark side of the family. In it is the spiritual counsel of Father Zossima ("Love is a harsh and dreadful thing") and the disciple and younger Karamazov brother, Alyosha. The soul of Russian spirituality can be found here as a healing, cauterizing fire. The spiritual elder Zossima says:

> What a book the Bible is, what a miracle, what strength is given with it to man! It is like a mould cast of the world and man and hu-

man nature, everything is there, and a law for everything for all the ages. And what mysteries are solved and revealed! God raises Job again, gives him wealth again. Many years pass by, and he has other children and loves them. But how could he love those new ones when those first children are no more, when he has lost them? Remembering them, how could he be fully happy with those new ones, however dear the new ones might be? But he could, he could. It's the great mystery of human life that old grief passes gradually into quiet, tender joy. The mild serenity of age takes the place of the riotous blood of youth. I bless the rising sun each day, and, as before, my heart sings to meet it, but now I love even more its setting, its long slanting rays and the soft, tender, gentle memories that come with them, the dear images from the whole of my long, happy life—and over all the Divine Truth, softening, reconciling, forgiving! My life is ending, I know that well, but every day that is left me I feel how earthly life is in touch with a new infinite, unknown, but approaching life, the nearness of which sets my soul quivering with rapture, my mind glowing and my heart weeping with joy.

George Eliot's *Middlemarch* (1871/1999) discusses the clash of professional talent and the community in the disastrous choices of Dr. Tertius Lydgate. Embedded in the grand architecture of a great novel, the story is about the social destruction of a gifted professional embroiled in unmanageable relationships that dry up his creativity. As to the ordinary and frail efforts to find peace in a loving family, Eliot's conclusion to the novel sings the praises of people such as her protagonist Dorothea Brooke and, really, we hope, of people such as us:

> But the effect of her being on those around her was incalculably diffusive, for the growing good of the world is partly dependent on unhistoric acts, and that things are not so ill with you or me as they might have been is half owing to the number who lived faithfully a hidden life and rest in unvisited tombs.

Finally, my old pastor used to say that if the minister dies with his or her boots on, the funeral will be crowded. Well, his was crowded, but not just because he died in his boots. His grave is visited often and I am one of the thankful people who go because I know that because of him "things are not so ill" with me as they might have been. He taught me and others how to love, not only among the ruins, but in the shadow of our humanity loved by God.

References

Alford, Helen and Naughton, Michael (2001). *Management As if Faith Mattered, Christian Social Principles in the Modern Organization*. Notre Dame, IN: University of Notre Dame Press.

Bernanos, Georges (1937). *Diary of a Country Priest*. New York: Macmillan Co.

The Bible (The New Oxford Annotated with the Aprocryphal/Deuterocanonical Books, New Revised Standard Edition) (1991). Oxford, England: Oxford University Press.

Buber, Martin (1923/1971). *I and Thou*. Repr. New York: Scribner's.

Bunyan, John (1684/1966). *The Pilgrim's Progress*. Repr. New York: Oxford Press.

Dostoevsky, Fyodor (1855/1992). *The Brothers Karamazov*. Repr. New York: Random House.

Dunne, John Gregory (1977). *True Confessions*. New York: Simon and Schuster.

Eliot, George (1871/1999). *Middlemarch*. Repr. New York: W.W. Norton.

Eliot, T. S. (1971). *The Complete Poems and Plays*. New York: Harcourt, Brace, and World.

Gallup Organization (2005). "How Important Is Religion in Your Own Life?" "At the Present Time On the Whole Do You Think Religion Is Increasing Its Influence or Losing?" "Are You Satisfied with the Current Moral and Ethical Climate?" Princeton, NJ: The Gallup Organization.

Gandhi, M.K. (1932). *From Yeravda Mandir (Letters to the Ashram)*. Ahmedabad, India: Navajivan Publishing House.

Greenleaf, Robert K. (1977). *Servant Leadership: A Journey into the Nature of Legitimate Power and Greatness*. Indianapolis, IN: The Greenleaf Center for Servant-Leadership.

Howe, Reuel (1963). *The Miracle of Dialogue*. New York: The Seabury Press.

Kelly, Thomas (1996). *A Testament to Devotion*. New York: HarperCollins.

Kieslowski, Krysztov (1988). *The Decalogue*. Chicago, IL: Facets Video (DVD).

Kieslowski, Krysztov (1993). *Blue*. Burbank, CA: Buena Vista Home Video.

LeSaux, Henri (Abhishiktananda) (1967). *Prayer.* New Delhi, India: ISPCK.

Lewis, C.S. (1950/2000). *The Chronicles of Narnia.* Repr. New York: HarperCollins.

Lopez, Donald (1999). *Prisoners of Shangri-La: Tibetan Buddhism and the West.* Chicago, IL: University of Chicago Press.

Loyola, Ignatius (2000). *Spiritual Exercises.* New York: Vintage Press.

Merton, Thomas (1949/1987). *Seeds of Contemplation.* Repr. New York: New Directions.

Merton, Thomas (1962/1972). *New Seeds of Contemplation.* Repr. New York: New Directions.

Merton, Thomas (1966). *Conjectures of a Guilty Bystander.* New York: Doubleday.

Merton, Thomas (1996). *Contemplative Prayer.* New York: Doubleday.

Montaldo, Jonathan and Hart, Patrick (1999). *The Intimate Merton: His Life from His Journal.* New York: HarperCollins.

Newman, John Henry (1899). "Christian Sympathy." *Plain and Parochial Sermons, V.* (pp. 126-127). London: Longmans, Green, and Co.

Newman, John Henry (1961). *On Consulting the Faithful in Matters of Doctrine.* New York: Sheed and Ward.

Newman, John Henry (1990). *Via Media.* Oxford, England: Oxford University Press.

Norris, Kathleen (1993). *Dakota: A Spiritual Geography.* New York: First Mariner.

Norris, Kathleen (1996). *The Cloister Walk.* New York: Riverhead.

Oakley, Francis and Russett, Bruce (2004). *Governance, Accountability, and the Future of the Catholic Church.* New York: Continuum.

Palmer, G.E.H., Sherrard, Philip, and Ware, Kallistos (Trans., 1995). *The Philokalia: The Complete Text.* Vol. 4. London: Faber and Faber Limited.

Pope John Paul II (1995). *That All May Be One (Ut Unum Sint).* Boston: Pauline.

Pope Paul VI (1996). *Paths of the Church (Ecclesiam Suam).* Boston: Pauline.

Report on the Crisis of the Catholic Church in the United States (2003). Washington, DC: United States Conference of Catholic Bishops.

Styron, William (1979/1992). *Sophie's Choice.* Repr. New York: Vintage.

Styron, William (1990/1992). *Darkness Visible: A Memoir of Madness.* Repr. New York: Vintage.

Teresa of Avila (1979). *The Interior Castle.* New York: Paulist Press.

Tolkien, J.R.R. (1954/2005). *The Lord of the Rings.* Repr. New York: Houghton Mifflin.

The Upanishads (trans. Juan Mascaro) (1965). New York: Penguin.

Vanier, Jean (1989). *Community and Growth.* New York: Paulist Press.

von le Fort, Gertrude (1954). *The Song of the Scaffold.* New York: Doubleday Image.

Warren, Rick (2002). *The Purpose-Driven Life.* Grand Rapids, MI: Zondervan.

Warren, Rick (1995). *The Purpose-Driven Church.* Grand Rapids, MI: Zondervan.

Welch, John (1982). *Spiritual Pilgrim: Carl Jung and Teresa of Avila.* New York: Paulist Press.

Index

Holocaust survivors, 34-35
Homosexuals, 64-65
Howe, Reuel, 33, 69
Human nature, 3-4

I and Thou, 33, 69
Incarnational side, ministry, 3
Interior Castle, 70
Intimate Merton, The, 70

Kekoa, Liz, 21-22, 24-25
Kelly, Thomas R., 70
Kieslowski, Krzysztof, 72

L'Arche, 68
Law, overuse of, 43
Lawyers, 41-45
Leadership, 55-60
LeSaux, Henri, 71
Letters to the Ashram, 71
Lewis, C.S., 67
Lopez, Donald, 71
Lord of the Rings, 67
Love, expressing, 63-64
Loyola, Ignatius, 71
Lydgate, Tertius, 73

Majority rule, 56
Managing As if Faith Mattered . . ., 68-69
Merton, Thomas, 70
Middlemarch, 73
Ministry
   light for, 60
   shadow side of, 2-3
Miracle of Dialogue, 33, 69
Monasticism, 51
Monette, Paul, 65
Montaldo, Jonathan, 70
Murder in the Cathedral, 14, 15

Natural sin, 65
Naughton, Michael, 45, 68-69
New Seeds of Contemplation, 70
Newman, John Henry, 35-36, 71-72
Norris, Kathleen, 70
Nouwen, Henri, 35

Oakley, Franklin, 72
Oliver, Mary, 71
On Consulting the Faithful in Matters of Doctrine, 71-72

Parents, 61-62
Path's of the Church (Ecclesiam Suam), 69
Peace, 38-39
Penalties, overuse of, 43
Perfectionism, 28
Philokalia, 70
Pilgrim's Progress, The, 67-68
Pius XII, 57
Pope John Paul II, 72
Pope John XXIII, 57
Pope Paul VI, 69
Poulenc, Francis, 68
Poustinia, 47
Power, 26
Prayer, 71
Prisoners of Shangri-La, 71
Professionalism, 28
Psalm 22, 15-18
Purpose-Driven Church, The, 71
Purpose-Driven Life, The, 71

Report on the Crisis of the Catholic Church in the United States, 69
Retreats, 47-50
Rock Hill, SC, 42, 55-56
Roles, 3, 22
Rule of St. Benedict, The, 71
Russett, Bruce, 72

Order a copy of this book with this form or online at:
http://www.haworthpress.com/store/product.asp?sku=5157

GRIEF, LOSS, AND DEATH
The Shadow Side of Ministry

_____in hardbound at $19.95 (ISBN-13: 978-0-7890-2414-5; ISBN-10: 0-7890-2414-4)

_____in softbound at $10.95 (ISBN-13: 978-0-7890-2415-2; ISBN-10: 0-7890-2415-2)

Or order online and use special offer code HEC25 in the shopping cart.

COST OF BOOKS_____

POSTAGE & HANDLING_____
(US: $4.00 for first book & $1.50
for each additional book)
(Outside US: $5.00 for first book
& $2.00 for each additional book)

SUBTOTAL_____

IN CANADA: ADD 7% GST_____

STATE TAX_____
(NJ, NY, OH, MN, CA, IL, IN, PA, & SD
residents, add appropriate local sales tax)

FINAL TOTAL_____
(If paying in Canadian funds,
convert using the current
exchange rate, UNESCO
coupons welcome)

☐ BILL ME LATER: (Bill-me option is good on
US/Canada/Mexico orders only; not good on
jobbers, wholesalers, or subscription agencies.)

☐ Check here if billing address is different from
shipping address and attach purchase order and
billing address information.

Signature_____

☐ PAYMENT ENCLOSED: $_____

☐ PLEASE CHARGE TO MY CREDIT CARD.

☐ Visa ☐ MasterCard ☐ AmEx ☐ Discover
☐ Diner's Club ☐ Eurocard ☐ JCB

Account # _____

Exp. Date_____

Signature_____

Prices in US dollars and subject to change without notice.

NAME_____

INSTITUTION_____

ADDRESS_____

CITY_____

STATE/ZIP_____

COUNTRY_____ COUNTY (NY residents only)_____

TEL_____ FAX_____

E-MAIL_____

May we use your e-mail address for confirmations and other types of information? ☐ Yes ☐ No
We appreciate receiving your e-mail address and fax number. Haworth would like to e-mail or fax special
discount offers to you, as a preferred customer. **We will never share, rent, or exchange your e-mail address
or fax number.** We regard such actions as an invasion of your privacy.

Order From Your Local Bookstore or Directly From
The Haworth Press, Inc.
10 Alice Street, Binghamton, New York 13904-1580 • USA
TELEPHONE: 1-800-HAWORTH (1-800-429-6784) / Outside US/Canada: (607) 722-5857
FAX: 1-800-895-0582 / Outside US/Canada: (607) 771-0012
E-mail to: orders@haworthpress.com

For orders outside US and Canada, you may wish to order through your local
sales representative, distributor, or bookseller.
For information, see http://haworthpress.com/distributors

(Discounts are available for individual orders in US and Canada only, not booksellers/distributors.)

PLEASE PHOTOCOPY THIS FORM FOR YOUR PERSONAL USE.
http://www.HaworthPress.com   BOF06